T0385463

PRACTICING FOOD STUDIES

Practicing Food Studies

Edited by
Amy Bentley,
Fabio Parasecoli, *and*
Krishnendu Ray

Foreword by Marion Nestle

NEW YORK UNIVERSITY PRESS
New York

NEW YORK UNIVERSITY PRESS
New York www.nyupress.org

Please contact the Library of Congress for Cataloging-in-Publication data.

ISBN: 9781479828081 (hardback)
ISBN: 9781479828098 (paperback)
ISBN: 9781479828111 (library ebook)
ISBN: 9781479828104 (consumer ebook)

This book is printed on acid-free paper, and its binding materials are chosen for strength and durability. We strive to use environmentally responsible suppliers and materials to the greatest extent possible in publishing our books.

Manufactured in the United States of America

10 9 8 7 6 5 4 3 2 1

Also available as an ebook

CONTENTS

FOREWORD

Interdisciplinarity and the Making of a Public Intellectual

MARION NESTLE

I view my professional identity as that of a public health nutritionist and food studies scholar. From this perspective, the most important global problems are food insecurity and its resulting hunger and malnutrition (affecting about one billion people); obesity and its health consequences (more than two billion), and the environmental effects of food production and consumption patterns (everyone on the planet) (FAO et al. 2019; Intergovernmental Panel on Climate Change 2019). These problems result in large part from inadequately functioning food systems, the current term for everything a food encounters from production, distribution, and sales to preparation, consumption, and waste (FAO et al. 2019; Nesheim, Oria, and Yih 2015). Understanding how food systems influence these problems necessarily requires a review of the history of their development, knowledge of their social, economic, political, and behavioral determinants, and at least some familiarity with nutrition science—how the intake of food, nutrients, and energy affects health.

I am not alone in prioritizing these problems and identifying their roots in dysfunctional food systems. In 2019, two interdisciplinary committees commissioned by the *Lancet*, a medical journal published in Great Britain, issued lengthy reports recommending specific personal dietary changes as well as actions by governments, the food industry, and civil society to do "triple duty" and address all three problems simultaneously. The EAT-Lancet Commission on Healthy Diets from Sustainable Food Systems recommended a "Great Food Transformation" to diets that contain half the amount of meat currently consumed in industrialized societies but twice the servings of fruits and vegetables (Willet et al. 2019). The Lancet Commission on the Global Syndemic of

Obesity, Undernutrition, and Climate Change called for government regulations along with an international policy framework to achieve healthier and more sustainable diets based on food systems thinking (Swinburn et al. 2019).

Because the influence of the food industry on personal dietary choices and public policy has been the focus of my research and teaching since the mid-1990s, I particularly appreciated the force and clarity of *Lancet*'s global syndemic report. That commission positioned the linked epidemics of hunger, obesity, and climate change as rooted in "consumptogenic" (i.e., capitalist, neoliberal) economic systems that overly empower food corporations, encourage privatization of public goods, permit for-profit companies to externalize the health and environmental costs of food production, and allow governments to be so effectively captured that they are unwilling or unable to curtail the risks generated by unregulated corporate power. The commission explained current policy inertia as the result of strong food industry opposition in the context of weak governance and weak civil society.

I was particularly impressed by the commission's suggestions for rebalancing power in the food system. It not only called for ending subsidies and tax breaks for food corporations but also for regulations to require corporations to pay the externalized costs of what they produce, to stop them from fighting public health measures, to keep them out of public policy decisions, to ensure that they disclose conflicts of interests and political donations, and to hold them fully accountable for the damage they cause to health, the environment, and democratic institutions. Although I have been suggesting measures like these for years, I had never previously seen them issued by a major international report. I considered this *Lancet* commission's food systems approach to be groundbreaking.

TRANSITIONS IN THINKING

I did not always understand or appreciate the importance of considering food systems as a means to analyze problems in nutrition and health. I began my career as a basic scientist, but over the years shifted interests to nutrition, public health, and, eventually, to food systems. In retrospect, I can explain these shifts most easily as having occurred in three distinct but somewhat overlapping stages.

Transition 1: Microbiology to molecular biology to nutrition. I was always interested in food, but at the time I began college, I was aware of only two options for studying it: agriculture and dietetics. Agriculture was out; I was a city girl and did not understand its importance for human health until much later. Instead, I went to the University of California Berkeley in the mid-1950s as a dietetics major, but I dropped that major immediately. The program required the same basic chemistry course taken by biology and premedical students; I found science more compelling. I became a science major and eventually completed my degree in bacteriology, but most of my friends were studying social sciences and humanities. I wanted to know what they knew. I took a course in public health and advanced courses in sociology, political science, and history. After graduation, I worked as a laboratory technician in Berkeley's school of public health, left that to start a family, did graduate study in molecular biology at Berkeley, and followed that with postdoctoral work in biochemistry and developmental biology at Brandeis University.

As a postdoctoral fellow, I was forced to recognize my inability to manage the time demands of bench science while raising two children. I left the laboratory and took an instructor's position in the Brandeis biology department, where I ran its basic laboratory course but also taught cell and molecular biology. This was in the early 1970s when students were pressing universities for liberalizing changes; Brandeis students wanted more courses in human biology. In 1975, I was given the choice of developing a new course in human physiology or human nutrition. I picked nutrition.

I was intrigued by nutrition science; it seemed refreshingly new. Linus Pauling's *Vitamin C and the Common Cold* (1970) was on bestseller lists. So was Frances Moore Lappé's *Diet for a Small Planet* (1971), which noted the environmental effects of eating meat and the health and planetary benefits of largely plant-based diets. The food advocacy group Center for Science in the Public Interest had been established in 1971; it had just published *Food for People, Not for Profit* (1975), a collection of articles on a broad range of food and nutrition topics, from agriculture to public health. The historian Geoffrey Barraclough, then at Brandeis, had just published articles in the *New York Review of Books* on the world food crisis and on the politics of food (1975a, 1975b). I was curious to know the extent to which science supported the ideas in these writings. Along with a basic nutrition textbook, I assigned these works as readings in that first course.

I experienced teaching this material as something like falling in love and never looked back. Whereas undergraduate biology majors could not easily read and critique original research in scientific journals, they could dive into nutrition research, and enthusiastically. Using nutrition as an entry point facilitated the teaching of basic biology, digestive physiology, and metabolism. Questions about the role of food in society and the societal factors influencing food production and choice arose naturally from students' personal experience with diets, were integral to the scientific discussions, and complemented them. I enjoyed teaching about the uncertainties of nutrition science, the challenges involved in determining what people eat, the need to put science in its societal context, and, of course, the dependence of nutrients on their food sources.

Transition 2: Basic nutrition science to clinical nutrition to public health nutrition. Much of that first course focused on individual nutrients, their roles in physiology and metabolism, and their food sources. Students asked for a more advanced course, and I taught a second semester of nutrient-based science in the spring of 1976. That fall, I moved to the University of California San Francisco (UCSF) to teach nutrition to medical students. For the next several years, I gave lectures, taught courses, and ran programs about the role of diet in health, diets for specific clinical conditions, parenteral and enteral nutrition, and nutrition counseling. My teaching dealt mainly with the physiological consequences of malnutrition, hunger, and obesity but necessarily drew on social, economic, political, and behavioral aspects when dealing with the causes of these conditions. But I was doing this teaching without a license; I had no formal training in nutrition. When the lack of credentials contributed to the loss of my job at UCSF, I was advised to obtain a master's degree in public health nutrition and did so.

At the time, I did not fully understand why I needed that credential. I held a doctorate and had just published my first book, *Nutrition in Clinical Practice* (1985), which summarized the material I had been teaching for the past decade. But I soon learned what I had been missing. Public health is about how forces in society determine the health risks of populations; it is about groups more than individuals, prevention of illness rather than treatment, and societal rather than personal determinants of health. It is highly sensitive to socioeconomic inequities and therefore is highly democratic. It fit my way of thinking. I especially appreciated the field work. I spent the year working part time with San Francisco's Coalition of Homeless Shelter Providers. I was able to meet the full-time summer fieldwork requirement through teaching a course in Shanghai and doing a research project on urban malnutrition for the US Agency for International Development in Bangkok and Jakarta.

By the end of this year of public health training, I knew that I wanted to work in nutrition policy as a means to improve the dietary practices of individuals and populations. I moved to Washington, DC, to work in the US Office of Disease Prevention and Health Promotion with primary responsibility for managing the writing and production of the first (and, as it turned out, only) *Surgeon General's Report on Nutrition and Health*, published in 1988 (DHHS 1988). After two years on a steep learning curve about how government nutrition programs do and do not work, I left to take a position as chair of what was then the Department of Home Economics and Nutrition at New York University.

Transition 3: Nutrition to foods to food politics and food systems. When I arrived at NYU in the late 1980s, the department housed programs in home economics, of course, but its stronger programs were in dietetics and food service management. These offered a variety of beginning and advanced courses about food and food preparation. The department also offered a small continuing education program of cuisine classes taught by local chefs. When, as I will explain, the opportunity arose to develop programs in food studies, the department could base the new programs on courses already in place.

I trace my interest in food politics to a meeting I attended at the National Cancer Institute in the early 1990s. My talk was about diet and cancer risk, but most of the other speakers spoke about cigarette smoking. Several showed slides of cigarette marketing, especially focused on people in developing countries and on children. I left that meeting thinking that nutritionists should be paying far more attention to the marketing of soft drinks and junk foods (what we now call ultra-processed foods). I began writing articles about the ways food companies influence food choices and health, and in the late 1990s I used that material as the basis for *Food Politics* (2002) and *Safe Food* (2003).

In 2006, the food studies faculty added a concentration in food systems to the existing concentration in food culture (more about the history of the department's food studies program below). Early the next year, for a talk at a conference on small farms at Oregon State University, I showed a slide labeled "Food System" to illustrate links between agriculture, food, nutrition, and public health as a basis for understanding personal dietary choices and food policy. I have used a version of that slide in nearly every subsequent talk to explain the interconnectedness of food issues. Since my retirement from NYU in 2017, I have continued to teach short courses titled *Food Systems Policy and Politics*, specifically aimed at integrating concepts derived from science, social and behavioral sciences, economics, and public health to help students understand and critically evaluate current issues related to food production and consumption.

METHODOLOGICAL APPROACHES

As a scientist, I was trained to use and value empiricism. Bench science involves formulating hypotheses, testing the hypotheses using appropriate laboratory techniques, controlling for potentially confounding alternative explanations of results, endlessly repeating experiments to confirm the results, and diligently keeping records of how the testing was done. As a graduate student, I isolated an enzyme that split DNA. To find out where the splits occurred, I had to develop a new method for separating the cleaved products, which I described in my first published paper (Nestle and Roberts 1968). But in my graduate training, what mattered was the research question—its importance, not how it was answered. Methods had to be appropriate but were decidedly secondary to whether the research question was "interesting." Except for those who were developing new methods, scientists who focused on "how" rather than "what for" were viewed as engaged in less interesting work. The kind of science that I was doing gave unambiguous results; the experiments either worked or did not and required no statistical tests for interpretation—a situation markedly different from that of research on food choices, dietary intake, and the effects of specific foods and diets on health.

For such questions, the scientific method has only limited applicability. Because humans are not experimental animals, vary in genetics, eat diets of great complexity, and vary in lifestyles, nutrition research is fraught with uncontrollable confounders and susceptibility to error. The principal quantitative methods for determining what people eat depend on individual self-reports of consumption over twenty-four hours or, for epidemiological studies of populations, through food-frequency questionnaires probing intake of specific foods for the last week, month, or year. Self-reported intake is well established to be subject to selective memory lapses, exaggeration of intake of supposedly good foods, and minimization of intake of supposedly bad foods, along with a 30 percent or greater underestimation of caloric intake. The results of nutrition studies often show only small differences that require careful interpretation, usually through the use of statistical tests to decide whether the differences could have occurred by chance. These flaws, long understood by nutrition scientists who interpret their results as best they can, have recently been rediscovered by statisticians who argue that because such methods sometimes lead to implausible results, nutrition research requires a total overhaul (Ioannidis 2013, 2018). Such critics, however, do not suggest meaningful methodologic alternatives.

Qualitative methods are often better for understanding why people choose particular foods or diets and how to promote dietary change. When I write about contemporary food politics, I find it useful to draw on the qualitative methods of history, psychology, economics, political science, and sociology to evaluate current government documents, newspaper accounts, and other components of non-peer reviewed "gray" literature. I know many scientists who view qualitative methods as non-research and multidisciplinary fields to be non-disciplines; they consider the work produced by such methods and fields as merely descriptive. But I have found qualitative methods to be essential for explaining the influence of food marketing on food choice (*Food Politics*, 2002, 2007, 2013) and, more recently, the influence of food industry funding on the outcome of nutrition research (Nestle 2015, 2018).

WRITING FOR A PUBLIC AUDIENCE

Nutrition research is necessarily aimed at identifying diets that maximize health and longevity; it is necessarily applied. But because the results of nutrition research usually require interpretation, their implications for personal food choice are not always straightforward. In teaching about diet and disease risk, I have always tried to be as clear as possible about the applications of nutrition research—its implications for personal dietary choices and public policy. As a lecturer in nutrition at UCSF, I received requests from its public relations office to answer questions from reporters. In the early 1980s, I did a series of thirteen segments on nutrition and health for a public television program, *Over Easy*, aimed at older viewers (one segment, for example, was with the *New York Times* food writer Craig Claiborne and Bay Area chef Narsai David). I wrote reviews of books about nutrition and health for the magazine *Medical Self-Care*. In Washington, DC, I wrote or rewrote most of the 1988 *Surgeon General's Report on Nutrition and Health*, which was meant to be understood well enough to inform nutrition policy. By the early 1990s, I had become a frequent source for reporters writing stories about nutrition issues. I considered dealing with their questions to be part of my university community service and well worth whatever time it took for them to get the facts right and interpret them reasonably.

To reach a wide audience, I have written an almost daily blog since 2007. From 2008 to 2013, I wrote a monthly food column for the *San Francisco Chronicle*. Although I try to make all of my books accessible to educated readers, I have written four specifically for a more general audience. *What to Eat* appeared in 2006; in it, I used supermarket aisles as an organizing device to address a wide range of food issues. In collaboration with Sara Thaves of the Cartoon Bank, I wrote the text of *Eat, Drink, Vote*, a book displaying more than two hundred cartoons drawn by artists that she represented (2013). In 2020, I published a book of short essays about the food politics of individual diets, communities, and the world, constructed as answers to questions posed by Kerry Trueman (*Let's Ask Marion*). And in 2022, the University of California Press published my memoir of all this, *Slow Cooked: An Unexpected Life in Food Politics*.

I want to reach general audiences. I believe that it is good for society, for the planet, and for democracy to ensure that everyone, regardless of income, race, class, gender, or age, is able to choose and consume diets that are healthier and more sustainable. People are confused about nutrition. I believe that helping to clear up that confusion is a worthwhile enterprise.

FOOD STUDIES AT NYU

I chaired what is now called the Department of Nutrition and Food Studies at NYU from 1988 to 2003. During that time, we developed programs in food studies to provide the kind of academic environment we would have chosen for ourselves from the beginning, had it existed. We were able to create this new field of study through a series of fortuitous circumstances.

From 1990 to 1995, I was often invited to attend and speak at international conferences organized by a Boston-based "culinary think tank," Oldways Preservation and Exchange Trust (Gifford and Baer-Sinnott 2006). Oldways' conferences brought together chefs, food writers, and academics to discuss the health and environmental value of traditional diets, particularly those of olive-growing Mediterranean countries (the group's chief sponsor was the International Olive Oil Council). At these conferences, I met talented chefs and food writers who told me of their deep interest in learning more about the history of food and its role in culture.

Boston University, urged by the chefs Julia Child and Jacques Pépin, had introduced a master's program in gastronomy in 1991, locating it within Metropolitan College, the university's continuing education division (Boston University). I wished that we could do something like that at NYU.

Before I arrived at NYU, the department's programs in food service management had evolved into—and were promoted as—programs in hotel management. I was concerned about the academic quality of that enterprise but was unable to do much about it. In 1995, a New York food consultant, Clark Wolf, offered help. He was well connected to the greater New York food community and put together an advisory committee composed of leading food producers, restaurateurs, chefs, food service managers, hotel managers, food journalists, writers, and editors along with some interested NYU professors in other departments. This committee reviewed the existing curricula and made one overriding suggestion: teach more about food. In response, we began working on curriculum revisions.

While those revisions were underway, the NYU administration decided to develop the equivalent of a hotel school within the School of

Continuing Education and called for transferring our food (and hotel) management programs to that school, an action that would reduce our tuition income by more than $1 million a year. When the dean asked what I wanted in return, I had a ready answer: "Food studies." The dean's response: "What's that?"

I knew that Boston University's gastronomy model would not work for NYU. We needed a title that would better reflect our purpose. NYU already offered many programs labeled "studies"—Africana studies, American studies, and Asian studies, for example, just in the "A's" alone. Feeling sorry for our plight, the dean took the risk that we would somehow be able to attract students to this new field, gave the department a new tenure line, and got the School of Continuing Education to pay for renovation of the department's 1950s home economics kitchen. Over the next nine months, we recruited Amy Bentley, an American studies historian, to develop the program, turned the kitchen into a modern food laboratory space, wrote proposals for new undergraduate, master's, and doctoral programs in food studies, and obtained the necessary approvals from the university and the New York State Board of Education.

One week after obtaining state approval, Marian Burros, a food writer for the *New York Times*, wrote about our program (1996). That very afternoon, prospective students came to our office holding clippings of the article, telling us that they had waited all their lives for this program. We had a class when our programs started in the fall of 1996.

Burros, who had been writing about the politics of food for many years, interviewed many sources for her story: me, Amy Bentley, and Clark Wolf but also a range of figures in the worlds of food and nutrition. Some expressed doubts. Burros quoted biochemistry professor John Suttie reflecting the attitude of many basic scientists that people trained in interdisciplinary subjects "are trained to do nothing." She also quoted Alice Waters, of the restaurant Chez Panisse in Berkeley, who objected that "the program needs real emphasis on the agriculture side. . . . The students should have to go out and grow tomatoes and harvest potatoes."

At the time, I was incredulous. NYU is decidedly urban. Were we supposed to be growing vegetables in Washington Square Park? But of course she was right in insisting that food studies be applied as well as theoretical. Ten years later, we introduced the concentration in food systems; we also filed the first of many petitions to the university for space to build a farm. In 2013, after years of dealing with one bureaucratic hurdle after another, we were able to break ground behind a landmarked I. M. Pei faculty-housing building to establish the department's now flourishing Urban Farm Laboratory (chapter 13 provides more detail on the Urban Farm Lab).

I must mention one additional fortuitous event: development of the NYU Library's food studies collection (which, I could not be more pleased to note, has been named in my honor). This began in the early 2000s when a professorial friend in California forwarded a notice she had been sent about the availability of a large collection of cookbooks belonging to Cecily Brownstone, then in her nineties and long retired from a forty-year career as food reporter for the Associated Press. Until then, the library had resisted collecting books about food on the grounds that they were "not scholarly" and "not of general academic interest." But a new curator of special collections, Marvin Taylor, thought it was the library's responsibility to support food studies programs and arranged for purchase of Brownstone's ten thousand or so books and five thousand pamphlets and food ephemera (Severson 2005). Taylor's active collecting program has resulted in a world-class library of about sixty-five thousand books on food and cooking, in constant use by NYU and other scholars from every imaginable field of study (NYU Libraries Special Collections and Archives).

What all this means is that the environment of NYU's food studies programs enables us to deal with critical problems in society, in my case, capitalism (which scares students), through the lens of food (which does not). Food studies unites and supports my interests in how food company marketing imperatives affect hunger, obesity, food production, and climate change and how to advocate for food systems that are healthier for people and the planet.

REFERENCES

Barraclough, Geoffrey. 1975a. "The Great World Crisis I." *New York Review of Books*, January 23. http://www.nybooks.com.

———. 1975b. "Wealth and Power: The Politics of Food and Oil." *New York Review of Books*, August 7 http://www.nybooks.com.

Boston University, Gastronomy Program History. https://sites.bu.edu.

Burros, Marian. 1996. "A New View on Training Food Experts." *New York Times*, June 19. https://www.nytimes.com.

Center for Science in the Public Interest. 1975. *Food for People, Not for Profit*. New York: Ballantine.

Department of Health and Human Services (DHHS). 1988. *The Surgeon General's Report on Nutrition and Health*. Publ. No. (PHS) 88–50210. Washington, DC: US Government Printing Office.

FAO, IFAD, UNICEF, WFP, and WHO. 2019. *The State of Food Security and Nutrition in the World 2019. Safeguarding against Economic Slowdowns and Downturns*. Rome: Food and Agricultural Organization of the United Nations. http://www.fao .org.

Gifford, K. Dun, and Sara Baer-Sinnott. 2006. *The Oldways Table: Essays & Recipes from the Culinary Think Tank*. Berkeley, CA: Ten Speed Press.

Intergovernmental Panel on Climate Change. 2019. *Climate Change and Land: An IPCC Special Report*. https://www.ipcc.ch/srccl/.

Ioannidis, John P. A. 2013. "Implausible Results in Human Nutrition Research." BMJ 347:f6698. doi: https://doi.org/10.1136/bmj.f6698.

———. 2018. "The Challenge of Reforming Nutritional Epidemiologic Research." *Journal of the American Medical Association* 320 (10): 969–70.

Lappé, Frances Moore. 1971. *Diet for a Small Planet* New York: Ballantine.

Lee, Robert D., and David C. Nieman, 1993. *Nutritional Assessment*. Madison, WI: Brown & Benchmark.

Nesheim, Malden C., Maria Oria, and Peggy Tsai Yih, eds. 2015. *A Framework for Assessing Effects of the Food System*. Washington, DC: National Academies Press.

Nestle, Marion. 1985. *Nutrition in Clinical Practice*. Greenbrae, CA: Jones Medical Publications.

———. 2002. *Food Politics*. Berkeley: University of California Press.

———. 2003. *Safe Food*. Berkeley: University of California Press.

———. 2006. *What to Eat*. New York: North Point Press.

———. 2013. *Eat, Drink, Vote: An Illustrated Guide to Food Politics*. New York: Rodale.

———. 2015. *Soda Politics: Taking on Big Soda (and Winning)*. New York: Oxford University Press.

———. 2018. *Unsavory Truth: How Food Companies Skew the Science of What We Eat*. New York: Basic Books. 2022. *Slow Cooked: An Unexpected Life in Food Politics*. Oakland: University of California.

Nestle, Marion, and Walden K. Roberts. 1968. "Separation of Ribonucleosides and Ribonucleotides by a One-Dimensional Paper Chromatographic System." *Analytical Biochemistry* 22:349–351.

Nestle, Marion, and Kerry Trueman. 2020. *Let's Ask Marion: What You Need to Know about the Politics of Food, Nutrition, and Health*. Oakland: University of California Press.

New York University Libraries. Food Studies: Special Collections and Archives. https:// guides.nyu.edu/.

Pauling, Linus. 1970. *Vitamin C, the Common Cold, and the Flu*. San Francisco: W. H. Freeman.

Severson, Kim. 2005. "Want That on Rye, or in Writing?" *New York Times*, November 4. www.nytimes.com.

Singer, Merrill. 2009. *Introducing Syndemics: A Critical Systems Approach to Public and Community Health*. New York: Wiley.

Swinburn, Boyd A., Vivica I. Kraak, Steven Allender, Vincent J. Atkins, Phillip I. Baker, Jessica R. Bogard, Hannah Brinsden, et al. 2019. "The Global Syndemic of Obesity, Undernutrition, and Climate Change." *Lancet* 393 (10173): 791–846.

Willett, Walter, Johan Rockström, Brent Loken, Marco Springmann, Tim Lang, Sonja Vermeulen, Tara Garnett, et al. 2019. "Food in the Anthropocene: The EAT-Lancet Commission on Healthy Diets from Sustainable Food Systems." *Lancet* 393 (10170): 447–92.

Practicing Food Studies

An Introduction

FABIO PARASECOLI AND AMY BENTLEY

What is food studies? How do scholars, practitioners, and students with very different backgrounds interact in this interdisciplinary—and increasingly transdisciplinary—space? And what is food studies at New York University, one of the first departments in the world dedicated to this field? These are some of the questions that prompted us to begin working on this collective volume. We examine the food studies program at New York University as a specific case within food studies, as an expanding domain of research with historical, cultural, and other antecedents. We explore the larger context in which they emerged in terms of intellectual history and sociology of knowledge. Tracing our own steps as scholars and practitioners in a relatively new field gave us the opportunity to reflect on how intellectual endeavors and academic initiatives are created and evolve as a response to institutional constraints and opportunities, the landscape of ideas, social movements, and public conversations. The volume presents a case study of academic fields at the intersection of applied and theoretical knowledge and practice that can help refocus and energize the humanities. Similar to the new field of digital humanities, NYU food studies is a useful example for how the humanities can remain relevant and engaged in problem solving while developing fruitful and exciting dialogues with other intellectual traditions and approaches.

The opportunity for this reflection arose as we thought through the origin of the department over two decades ago, its current state, and its future. This project also began in part to celebrate Marion Nestle, who founded the department in the 1990s when very few similar experiences like it existed (and many frankly thought the idea had no legs).

We also wanted to celebrate her well-deserved retirement, although in her capacity as professor emerita, she is as active as ever as a researcher, writer, and public speaker, remaining an important presence not only in the department but in the world of food. Her role in legitimizing food studies as a field of research and practice is widely recognized not only in academia but also by civil society.

As often happens, as we commenced this project, we were not fully aware of the intellectual and, in many cases, emotional adventures in store for us, as individuals and as a collective. We began by sending out a call to all faculty, former and current doctoral students, and a few interested others who over the years have interacted with us. While this collection of essays contains a few holes here and there, overall it is a fairly good representation of the scope and evolution of NYU food studies—and food studies as a field in general. In fact, we want to underline that this collection is not meant to suggest that NYU food studies is more relevant or more advanced than other programs now thriving both in the United States and around the world. We are also fully aware that important work is being developed by colleagues in departments that are not exclusively dedicated to food studies and in programs such as agricultural sciences, food design, and food-focused MBAs that, although strictly speaking do not adopt a food studies approach, contribute to the overall advancement of the field. In fact, this exploration of NYU food studies should be considered as the analysis of a specific case study within a much broader field. Knowledge is never produced in isolation, and it is crucial to better understand what factors may contribute to its emergence and development over time. We hope readers find these essays useful to reflect on their own experience of what food studies is and where it is going. As Jon Deutsch suggests in his essay, the first decade of food studies established it as a legitimate field within academia, while the second decade demonstrated that scholars who identified with it were able to produce interesting and important research across the humanities and social sciences, in a multidisciplinary dialogue with health scholars and professionals, as well as with the culinary arts. What will the future bring? How will food studies grow both as a field and as an active participant in the cultural, social, and political debates that are shaping our world?

Articulating a Common Language

These questions, although not yet fully articulated, loomed large in the development of this edited volume. Right from the start, participants had different points of view and approaches, reflecting personal histories, theoretical perspectives, and ideas of processes and end goals of the project. Given that we are a collection of individuals from different intellectual backgrounds, aligned in a department where nutrition (and previously public health) plays a crucial and visible role, it became necessary for us to reflect how our personal and collective work has been shaped and influenced, allowing us to exchange ideas and knowledge with each other, understand one another, and teach students coherently. We all come from a specific discipline or method (nutrition, public health, sociology, history, economics, or interdisciplinary fields such as American studies and food studies), but our work in some way goes beyond our narrower home disciplines. Thus, many of us would not necessarily "fit" in a traditional history or sociology department, for example.

For these reasons, we decided to come together in a workshop to identify the elements that we share as well as the characteristics that make us unique. During the four-hour workshop (held in the fall of 2019), participants worked collaboratively, following a structured process that was meant to generate some form of deliverables. It was uncomfortable for some, because we were asked to react quickly and to give immediate responses rather than taking our time to reflect (which is unusual for us, as academics). It was the first time that most of us had engaged in such an undertaking. We were aiming to build more on collective wisdom than on individual thoughts. We hoped that the workshop would be useful to come up with ideas and solutions that would not have emerged had we stuck to more familiar methods. As they say, there are no bad suggestions in brainstorming, and all participants tried their best to embrace this point of view, feeling free to offer ideas that may have sounded silly, unclear, or emotional and shrugging it off if they did not receive the feedback they expected.

The various activities we engaged in followed a methodology known as "design thinking," which has been developed in design but is now also widely used in business, marketing, and increasingly in academic research. In broad strokes, design thinking usually proceeds following the subsequent phases of exploration > gathering insights > ideation > prototyping > testing (Brown 2019; Lewrick, Link, and Leifer 2020). We went through a series of exercises that were meant to help us better focus on our understanding of the field in general but also, more practically, to generate a set of actionable ideas about the content and the structure of the volume that you are now reading and to provide a blueprint that the editors could use in guiding the writing process as we were getting ready to write our individual chapters.

The result of the workshop was both a snapshot of our identity as a department that helped us find a common language while writing our individual essays, and a more general reflection in the sociology of knowledge: How is knowledge produced in food studies? Which structures and dynamics underlie such production? What is the role of context and of the specific intellectual biographies of those involved? How is food studies as it is taught, researched, and practiced at New York University different from how it is approached at other institutions?

Through the design workshop, we realized that NYU food studies, similar to departments elsewhere, provides a sense of home. It constitutes a place for people on the margins of disciplines; at times, we have felt that other academics do not fully understand what we do or even dismiss our work. Food studies may be hard to define, as it does not have the structure of a discipline but rather points to a field that generates tensions between generalists and specialists. It lacks a coherent canon of scholarship, which many of us think is a good thing. It has generally derived from feminine domestic realms; as a case in point, the NYU food studies department used to be home economics.

Often there is the need to explain ourselves in ways that academics from other disciplines and fields do not have to. Some critics may feel we should be focusing on more "serious" topics. Our work may be viewed by some as trivial, elitist, too white, preachy, and narcissistic—too idealistic, without consideration of real-life constraints; too influenced by hipster frameworks and priorities.

However, through the workshop exercises and discussion, we realized that these critiques cause minimal worry. We take food seriously; we realize how crucial it is for both individuals and communities, at all scales and levels. While we all made our way to NYU food studies through different paths (some have purely academic training, others also have professional backgrounds in kitchens, food production, and journalism), that does not stop us from sharing an intellectual project. We may have different standpoints, but we often end up looking at the same set of issues.

Additionally, workshop discussions revealed that focusing exclusively on food may not provide the best solutions to food problems. We at times risk buying into an attitude that fixates on single issues with solutions that would magically redo the food system. We understand that there are contrasting values and goals regarding food, including pleasure (as a positive, creative element), consumerism (the food system is geared to produce more to the financial benefit of few), citizenship (what can we do to change the food system, to make it more just and secure?), and environmentalism (need for sustainability, and consideration of climate change). The complexity of overlapping issues combined with the tendency to zoom into more circumscribed and manageable matters can foster simplified "solutions" that can themselves create more complexity.

Finally, the workshop helped us become fully aware of real-world constraints on the production of purely intellectual and theoretical knowledge. Students come to us hoping to learn approaches and skills that they can apply in their professional lives, and we have to balance those demands with our research and theoretical interests; they also inevitably impact our teaching. Further, we feel that our work could or should have real-life applications. However, there are constant tensions and ongoing negotiations between the desire for a critique of the food system and the sometimes inevitable compromise with it, as we need to operate effectively in what is often referred to as "the real world." That said, we feel that we have to keep justice and equality as a goal also when dealing with the for-profit world.

What Is NYU Food Studies? Origins and Definitions

The workshop discussions and the work that followed them also led us to reflect on the development of food *studies* and our place in it as a department. Food studies as a field is generally defined as the multidisciplinary academic research and teaching of food grounded in the humanities and social sciences. Food studies has distinct and important antecedents in a number of disciplines, including anthropology, folklore, the *Annales* school—a brand of social history that focused on mundane everyday activities of medieval and early modern Europeans' lives—as well as sociology's world-systems theory, in which researchers recognized global flows of food commodities as central to their understanding of the emerging early modern world economy. Twentieth-century cultural anthropologists, including Audrey Richards, Claude Lévi-Strauss, Mary Douglas, and Marvin Harris, all wrote extensively and perceptively about the place of food in diverse cultures (Douglas 1966; Harris, 1975; Lévi-Strauss 2008; Richards 1939). In addition, folklorists also were instrumental in creating an academic space for the study of food. Donald Yoder, credited with coining the term *foodways*, for example, approached food as material culture in its vernacular settings in the United States (1972). These subdisciplines have long regarded the study of food as key to understanding cultures and societies and individuals' lives within them. Eating, after all, is much more than ingesting nutrients for biological survival; food plays a significant role in social relationships, is a highly symbolic element in religious rites, aids in developing and maintaining cultural distinctions, and assumes enormous significance in shaping individual identities. As food also helps to designate class, ethnicity, and gender, this kind of scholarship tends to be qualitative oriented, featuring questions that employ, for example, historical and cultural analysis, that critique the political economy of food, or that explore the meanings and uses of food. Borrowing from history, folklore, anthropology, sociology, and cultural studies, food studies tends to employ qualitative methods: cultural analysis, ethnography, case study, participant observation, interview, and archival data. It tends to be more focused on explaining the meanings and uses of phenomena—low-carb diets, for example—rather than proving their existence or their efficacy (Bentley 2004).

Food studies also owes a debt to the many biologists, food activists, nutritionists, economists, agrarian sociologists, and rural social scientists who have focused on the health aspects and production of food. More oriented toward the sciences/hard social sciences and quantitative methods, these scholars who study food production speak in terms of *food systems*, chains of institutions, processes, and peoples linking the production of food with its distribution. They tend to concentrate on the relations of food production to economics, the environment, and human nutrition yet increasingly have recognized the importance of understanding food in its social, cultural, and historical contexts. The activist and scholarly work in the 1970s and 1980s of Columbia University nutrition professor Joan Dye Gussow, for example, drew attention to the worst excesses of industrial food manufacturing and its nutrition and health effects on Americans. One of her most important studies documented the heavy sugar cereal and candy advertising during Saturday morning children's cartoons, work that was instrumental in FTC regulation of minimally nutritious food during children's programming (1980). In many ways, the tension between those who focus on cultural issues and those who instead emphasize the centrality of systemic factors, between agency and structure, has been a constitutive feature of the field since its inception. Although at times a source of misunderstanding and debate, such tension is also extremely productive, forcing us to look at food, as anthropologist Marcel Mauss would say, as a "total social fact":

> Phenomena are at once legal, economic, religious, aesthetic, morphological and so on. They are legal in that they concern individual and collective rights, organized and diffuse morality. . . . They are at once political and domestic, being of interest both to classes and to clans and families. . . . They are economic, for the notions of value, utility, interest, luxury, wealth, acquisition, accumulation, consumption and liberal and sumptuous expenditure are all present. (Mauss 1966, 76–77)

NYU food studies arose in the mid-1990s as part of this late-twentieth-century burgeoning academic interest in the cultural and social study of food. While food had always been a well-represented topic in the disciplines of anthropology and folklore, universities began to respond to growing interest with programs, courses, and academic research that focused on these groups and issues in urban contexts (which was slow in emerging). The emergence of such fields as women's studies, ethnic studies, material culture, and other programs that gave voice to the academic study of the everyday and the less powerful allowed for venues of discourse for food as a primary subject matter. In addition to concentration clusters and inter-department minors, stand-alone programs such as NYU food studies institutionally sanctioned food as a subject worthy of study (Bentley 2012).

NYU food studies is a distinct product of its location and history. Originally a home economics department, in the 1980s the NYU Home Economics Department changed its focus to become a nutrition program granting a registered dietitian (RD) credential as well as a food management program. This transformation was part of the larger trend of academic programs remaking themselves in response to the women's movement. With the arrival of Marion Nestle as chair (see her contribution to this collection), that focus began to further shift and evolve, as in 1996 when the management program was shed for a more academic multidisciplinary approach to food. Naming it "food studies" aligned the program of study to more of a humanities and social sciences bent.

As a program, we are immersed in different, overlapping dimensions that we try to articulate. We are primarily a BA and an MA program, with a small PhD program, in which multidisciplinarity works well, as it allows us to deliver rich, multifaceted knowledge and skills to our students. Over the years, we have become globally visible and relevant in the field of food studies, and we feel we participate in the shared effort to move the whole field forward, without considering our specific approach as a department as the only viable one.

While NYU food studies has been concretely shaped by NYU nutrition (and vice versa, as Lisa Sasson's essay in this collection attests), the relationship between our two programs, nutrition and food studies, has not been seamless. Food studies and nutrition are distinct programs of study that grew up with differing epistemologies. Nutrition emerged from the sciences: largely experimental, measuring and quantifying, discovering and understanding micronutrients, figuring out what the human body needs to first stay alive and second be healthy. Aligning itself with the sciences, research tends to be quantitative. Researchers however, have largely come to understand that their findings are reflective of a particular context, as being "healthy" means different things in different contexts and cultures. Food studies, by contrast, examines the historical, cultural, and sociopolitical aspects of food, primarily its consumption but more recently of production and processing as well. It is grounded in the "studies" end of academia, humanities, and soft social sciences, in contrast to the "sciences" end of the spectrum (Sobal 2002).

In part because of these epistemological differences, as food studies has matured we have seen the development of humanities-oriented fields that specifically critique the more empirical food and nutritional sciences. These include such offshoots as critical food studies, critical nutrition studies, critical eating studies, fat studies, and discard studies. Influenced by questions of power and inequality, and taking cues from science and technology studies and cultural studies, scholars have highlighted the discrepancies in and fallacies of objectivity and empiricism. While critiques of science are important and illuminating, our colleague Krishnendu Ray has offered a caution:

> We have to learn anew to attend to and respect the evidentiary rules for the sciences of objectivity in the study of food, such as biochemistry and nutrition, as much as climate change . . . to be careful what we challenge, on what basis, and how, because if we aid in tearing the social fabric of knowledge-making apart, then much of the alt-right's job would have been done, to sow radical doubt and turn knowledge production and information gathering as acts of warfare (2017).

At NYU food studies, we have assumed this more open approach to empiricism and science in large part because we daily interact with nutrition faculty and students, responding to their research and understanding their worldview, and in part because we have seen, especially through the work of Marion Nestle, the importance of critiquing United States food policy through a more empirically based view of science.

Methodological and Disciplinary Challenges

As a multidisciplinary field with topics that often cut across themes, there is a constant tension in food studies between keeping food at center, in and for itself, and using it as an entryway, a lens, or a mirror for other issues. Among other topics, we focus on culture, systems, sustainability, power and politics, labor, government, institutions, physical and emotional health. We also work at the intersections among them:

attempts at creating culinary heritage or canons; cultural politics that express themselves in debates about identity, authenticity, tradition, and appropriation; food as product and commodity; history. Materiality, sensoriality, and embodiment are fundamental to us: the aesthetics aspects of the issues we study are not an embellishment, they are central to what we do.

As we have abundantly made clear, food studies constantly deals with methodological issues, as there is an inherent tension when scholars and practitioners from various backgrounds find themselves working in the same space. Right now, we are multidisciplinary. Each of us has our own trajectory, methods, theories. That helps us avoid dogmatism; we do not have a unified theory we are faithful to. We rather share values and approaches. At least from the scholarly research and project point of view, we are working toward actual interdisciplinarity, where we can engage with each other in terms of methods, theories, and practices, with the goal of creating something that is not there yet.

That said, many of us are comfortable outside traditional disciplines or incorporating multiple methods. There are tensions between applied and theoretical knowledge, between scholarship and the quotidian, between teachers who are academics and students who may be aspiring for-profit professionals. In our work, we are expected to practice observation, analysis and critique, without turning our back on activism, advocacy, and other kinds of interventions. We deal with what designers may describe as "wicked problems," complex issues without univocal or unambiguous solutions, toward which stakeholders usually have contrasting needs, values, and goals and where interventions may have all sorts of unpredictable consequences.

In teaching and producing knowledge, we are often pulled between the desire to generate and impart practical skills and the need for discipline-based research, between applied knowledge and text-based scholarship, between the diffusion and production of knowledge through performativity and academic rigor, between storytelling, visual display, digital methods, and more traditional scholarship. It may be challenging to find a balance between the quantitative and empirical aspects of our work and the aspiration toward the qualitative and theoretical. On top of all this, we may encounter difficulties in relating to the hard sciences, which, however, are quite important (especially in a department that also hosts a nutrition program). We value our work with students, so pedagogy is a central concern.

Engagement with the Public Sphere

And that is only what we need to take into consideration within our academic world. However, we are constantly called to engage with the public sphere and popular culture. Our work frequently elicits interest because food studies is current, relatable, relevant, contextualized in history and current events, and concerned with ethical conundrums. Historically, food studies has valued engagement with the public and non-specialist audiences and collaborations with external partners as diverse as chefs, farmers, street food vendors, government agencies, and non-profit organizations.

When it comes to the specificities of food studies at New York University, we are undoubtedly shaped by our ecology, as we are part of a private university serving a public that is local and global in a broader sense than just geography, and of a school—Steinhardt—that prides itself for being at the intersection of theory and applied learning. We are influenced by our location in New York City, an important global media center. As a consequence, we are a networked space like few other places in food studies. As a result, we are open and outward looking, clear in our writing and arguments while connecting globally with researchers, theories, and debates that extend well beyond our location. Our capacity for multidisciplinary work, and our efforts toward interdisciplinarity, makes us better collaborators and increases our ability to build bridges with various sectors of civil society to achieve tangible results in shared projects.

This is what allows us to speak to journalists so readily, to work with public institutions, and to keep conventional jargon at a minimum. Some of us have become effective popularizers, in the best sense of the term, making our research available to the public outside of academia. We are involved in connections between the city and the rural world, between our nation and other countries, hence our interest and involvement in migration issues. To use an apt metaphor, we have to eat everything on our plate. If we don't eat it, we have to share it.

The Structure of the Book

The book begins with a foreword by Marion Nestle who tells the story of the department in her own voice. It seems to us the best way to open up a conversation that, while an assessment of the development and the current state of food studies, is also meant to acknowledge Nestle's work.

The remaining chapters are organized in three sections. The first, "Humanities and Social Sciences," looks at food studies from the point of view of various established disciplines and fields while reflecting on the challenges of multidisciplinarity from a theoretical and bibliographical point of view. The essays in this section illustrate experiences in the areas of history, sociology, poetry and literary studies, and performance studies. The second section, "Health, Nutrition, and the Culinary Arts," turns its attention on the department's engagement with individual and community health through the lenses of public health and nutrition, highlighting the relevance of food for both personal well-being and social dimensions such as justice, equity, and sustainability. It also focuses on the culinary arts and the role that recipes play in bringing food to the table, reminding us that the materiality of what we grow, process, prepare, and eat is central to food studies. Finally, the last section, "Technology and Applied Sciences," points to the potential of food studies to expand toward new areas such as design, network science, and library sciences and to provide the basis for technology startups and entrepreneurship. In the penultimate chapter, "Action Research and Social Engagement," several of us share experiences in our applied engagement with civil society and the community around us. Finally, Krishnendu Ray's concluding chapter presents some final thoughts regarding the pleasures and pitfalls of building an emerging field such as NYU food studies.

REFERENCES

Bentley, Amy. 2004. "The Other Atkins Revolution: Atkins and the Shifting Culture of Dieting." *Gastronomica* 4, no. 3 (August): 34–45.

———. 2012. "Sustenance, Abundance, and the Place of Food in United States Histories." In *Global Food Historiography: Researchers, Writers, & the Study of Food*, edited by Kyri Claflin and Peter Scholliers, 72–86. Oxford: Berg.

Brown, Tim. 2019. *Change by Design, Revised and Updated: How Design Thinking Transforms Organizations and Inspires Innovation.* New York: HarperCollins.

Douglas, Mary. 1966. *Purity and Danger: An Analysis of Concepts of Pollution and Taboo*. New York: Routledge.

Gussow, Joan. 1980. "Some Impractical Thoughts on Television & Nutritional Education." *Food Monitor* (November/December). Available at http://joansgarden.org.

Harris, Marvin. 1998. *Good to Eat: Riddles of Food and Culture*. Long Grove, IL: Waveland.

Lévi-Strauss, Claude. 2008. "The Culinary Triangle." In *Food and Culture: A Reader*, edited by Counihan and Van Esterik, 40–47. New York: Routledge.

Lewrick, Michael, Patrick Link, and Larry Leifer. 2020. *The Design Thinking Toolbox: A Guide to Mastering the Most Popular and Valuable Innovation Methods*. Hoboken, NJ: Wiley.

Mauss, Marcel. 1966. *The Gift: Forms and Functions of Exchange in Archaic Societies*. London: Cohen & West.

Ray, Krishnendu. 2017. "Uncertain Truths: On the Limits of the Critique of Globalization and the Sciences." *Food, Culture and Society* 20 (4): 563–68. doi: 10.1080/15528014.2017.1378497.

Richards, Audrey. 1939. *Land, Labour, and Diet in Northern Rhodesia: An Economic Study of the Bemba Tribe*. Oxford: Oxford University Press.

Sobal, Jeffrey. 2002. "Whither Food Studies?" NYU *Feast and Famine Thinking about Food*. January 31. Department of Nutrition, Food Studies and Public Health (copy in author's possession).

Yoder, Donald. 1972a. "Folk Cookery." In *Folklore and Folklife: An Introduction*, edited by Richard Dorson, 325–50. Chicago: University of Chicago Press.

———. 1972b. "Folk Costume." In *Folklore and Folklife: An Introduction*, edited by Richard Dorson, 295–324. Chicago: University of Chicago Press.

———. 1972c. "Folk Medicine." In *Folklore and Folklife: An Introduction*, edited by Richard Dorson, 191–216. Chicago: University of Chicago Press.

Humanities and Social Sciences

This first section looks at food studies from the point of view of established disciplines and fields while reflecting on the challenges of multidisciplinarity. The authors here examine food studies in relation to history, sociology, poetry and literary studies, and performance studies.

Food studies as an academic domain followed a similar trajectory to other multidisciplinary fields of study. Without detouring too much through the history of knowledge classification, for centuries universities have organized and classified knowledge into three main branches: natural sciences, social sciences, and humanities (with technology emerging as a practical extension of the natural sciences and performing and visual arts an extension of the humanities). Within these branches, knowledge was further organized via disciplines (economics, mathematics, philosophy), each with corresponding methods of data generation and analysis. By the twentieth century, these academic disciplines, largely products of the eighteenth and nineteenth centuries, felt constrained. Academic researchers found them inflexible, as problems such as environmental degradation or social inequality, for example, spanned multiple disciplines and methods. Departments and programs began to split disciplines into smaller fields, which often traversed a number of established disciplines employing multiple methods. These fields were often identified by the term *studies* (for the humanities/social sciences, primarily qualitative methods) or *sciences* (for social sciences/sciences, primarily quantitative methods). Food studies, of course, emerged in this space.

As detailed in the introduction, food studies is defined, first, as grounded in the humanities and social sciences. Multidisciplinary in its use of theory and methods, it leans toward the "studies" end as opposed to the "sciences" end of academic field spectrum. Faculty research, for example, tends to be qualitative, featuring questions that employ cultural or historical analysis or critique the political economy of food. Unlike the sciences, it is more focused on explaining the meanings and uses of phenomena rather than proving their "existence" or their efficacy. Second, NYU food studies takes food as a serious focus of academic study. While this is also true in most disciplines today, only in the last couple of decades has food been considered a legitimate topic of scholarly inquiry in the most traditional disciplines. Third, while grounded in humanities and social science methods and conventions, NYU food studies values and produces applied scholarship, engages with the public and non-specialist audiences, and collaborates with external partners.

The chapters in this section fall within the humanities (poetry/literary studies), social sciences (history, sociology) and interdisciplinary fields of studies (gender studies, performance studies). Each author understands their origin to be within these structures, though each seeks to contribute something new employing food as a focus.

1

History and Gender Studies

An Institutional Biography of NYU Food Studies

AMY BENTLEY

The early 2020s witnessed intense global transformational change. The brutal effects of the COVID-19 global pandemic shaped and amplified the continuing protests over the murders of George Floyd and Breonna Taylor (among others) as part of the Black Lives Matter movement, the ongoing #MeToo movement for gender equity, a profound rethinking of how we understand the founding of the United States and commemorate past leaders, and the dramatic curtailing of our democratic institutions by some in power. A significant feature of the COVID pandemic was the stark reality that people in food-service and food-production positions, deemed "essential workers" and thus more exposed to the virus, were largely people of color, a sizable number of whom are women. These store clerks, delivery people, restaurant workers, caregivers, and agriculture and food manufacturing employees toiled in potentially dangerous, mostly low-paid positions to make sure the rest of us were fed. It is important to acknowledge and express gratitude for their hard work and commitment. It also speaks to a central issue in this essay: women's long involvement in food work, mostly invisible and minimally paid, in both the private and public spheres.

There is a long history of fraught relations between gender and food, a relationship that elicits a broad range of emotions. Scholars studying food work and gender in foraging societies surmise that food labor was divided in large part as a result of biology and physiology. While clearly a generalization with ample room for exception, men, as a result of their larger muscle groups allowing on average more upper body strength, hunted or fished for bigger game. Women, partly due to their being the child bearers, usually stayed closer to home and engaged in a range of foraging duties, including fishing and netting smaller game, gathering plants, and planting and tilling (although recent scholarship has complicated this long-held template). Despite the symbolic power elicited by big game catches, researchers estimate that women's foraging netted some 70 percent of the total food supply. (Dahlberg 2009; Gibbons 2020; Haas et al. 2020; Hedenstiema-Jonson, et al. 2017; Newitz 2021). Further, anthropologist Richard Wrangham notes the universal norm across cultures of a hot meal in the evening, most often prepared by women (2010). Modern societies have been able to alter these habits and reassign these duties (to men or hired help, for example), but for most of human history this gendered labor of food has been the template.

While men have always been involved in food, it is women's particularly deep relationship and connection to food that is held up for closer examination here. In most societies, women have traditionally been responsible for preparing, producing, processing, serving, cleaning up, and often procuring meals for a household. Further, women's bodies are literally food for their infants as they grow in utero, and also afterward until the child is weaned. Nourishing and nurturing a child are intimately entwined, as it is in caregiving for the sick or elderly. While men have performed this work as well, for most of human history, its burden and blessings have fallen upon women. Modern currency-based economies and industrialization created even more pronounced household and family divisions of labor and more entrenched inequalities, as men's public-facing labor was more often paid, and women's domestic labor remained unpaid (Welter, 1966). Even when performing essentially the same cooking tasks, for example, men's work as professional chefs in the public sphere was compensated and held more prestige than women's cooking in the private domestic realm.

One can trace food studies' examination of women and food via sociology, anthropology, social history, women's and gender studies, and also nutritional sciences. Given the plethora of good scholarship on gender and food today, it is hard to remember that a generation or two ago, such topics were not considered serious enough for academic inquiry. How did we get from there to here? What are the factors that created the interest and focus? And what of the multidisciplinary scholarship and interest in gender and food in the twenty-first century? In this essay, I will examine my work vis-à-vis NYU food studies and will conclude with final thoughts about gender and food in the current moment.

NYU Food Studies and Gender:
A Program Shaped by Its Environment

As discussed in the introduction, NYU food studies is a product of certain constraints and realities, and through its evolution from home economics to a department of nutrition and food studies, the department retained its female centered aura and culture. This is for several reasons, the most obvious being that it had begun as a home economics department, a female dominated program if there ever was one. Second, the department studied food via the nutritional sciences, a field with its own unique history. While nutrition has antecedents in the traditionally male-dominated field of chemistry, nutrition programs with applied focus resulting in a registered dietitian credential, have always been more female-dominated—and in fact historically have been regarded as inferior by academia which privileges knowledge creation over knowledge dissemination, as well as theoretical knowledge over embodied knowledge (Shapiro, 1986). The NYU Nutrition and Food Studies Department was also housed in a school of education (now called the Steinhardt School of Culture, Education and Human Development) which has also been female dominated (similar to most education schools). Finally, NYU food studies focused its research and teaching on food as feeding and nourishing bodies, work that is less valued, especially in the public sphere, as Krishnendu Ray has discussed elsewhere (2016). It is also focused on the people who cook and serve the food, and the identities tied to it, as opposed to, for example, agricultural sciences. Food in this manner is about recipes, culture, feeding, identity—as opposed to economics, commodities, large-scale production, and so forth—another aspect of the program that locates it squarely within female territory.

As a food historian with an emphasis on gender, my work was already within this female-centered domain before I arrived at NYU food studies. My dissertation, a cultural history of World War II food rationing in the United States, examined the intersection of gender and the war and became a study of women's roles on the domestic home front in food procurement and preparation—essentially what Rosie the Riveter did when she left the factory and returned home to make dinner for her family. I began focusing on gender as the prime category of analysis but ended up most fascinated by the meanings and uses of food. As a graduate student in the late 1980s, I had come to the topic of women and food in history without real calculation. It seemed a perfectly natural topic; I was only peripherally aware that it was "new" or that it was regarded with some suspicion by more established older historians.

Just as women's and gender history has been a recent development, so has history focusing on food; in fact, the latter was largely made possible by the former. We study history for all kinds of reasons, most generally to avoid repeating the mistakes of the past (though we seem at best marginally successful at this) and to better understand who we are and where we come from. Studies show, for example, that children with a strong sense of family or community heritage and identity tend to perform better in school, contributing to more "grit" to weather through the tough times (Kelly 2012). History is also just interesting, as knowledge for knowledge's sake, and the history of food seems to resonate especially with the general public. It is a topic everyone has experience with, given that we all must eat, ideally several times a day, to survive. Even if people do not like to cook, think about, or even eat food, that aversion still registers as a force that makes people think and act. Thus, the absence of food, as well as its presence, becomes significant and meaningful.

That is where food history—cultural food history, to be more specific—comes in. It has only been fairly recent that such a topic in academia existed and was deemed legitimate beyond the women's pages in newspapers. Our understanding of history, as the written record of human activities and events, has expanded. A couple of generations ago, only certain subjects were thought important enough to be written about and studied, primarily institutional, economic and political events such as elections and battle tactics. Today, largely as a result of the late-twentieth-century turn to social and cultural history, there exists a broader range of topics also considered worthy of writing about, including the everyday lives of people "without a history"—women and children as well as men—as Eric Wolf termed it (1982). Advances in archeology and the study of material culture have helped to capture the histories of those without a written record. This in turn led to the academic examination of food—not just grain storage for civilizations and food as a commodity but the food ordinary people ate every day.

In the mid- to late 1980s, what academic work on food was available came from sociology and anthropology, disciplines that had been studying the social and cultural roles of food. In United States history, food was more of an afterthought, belonging more to labor history (meatpacking plants) and economic history (grain prices and the Great Depression/New Deal). Agricultural history existed, but scholarship focusing on the consumption of food was sparse, regarded as not important in current frameworks of historical knowledge, in part because the topic seemed too quotidian, too frivolous even, for *bona fide* academic history. The emerging field of women's history in the 1980s focused on writing women back into the main narratives of US history or discovering women's roles in the public sphere. Historians of gender were not much interested in the history of food, as it seemed too close to traditional domestic roles that women felt limited by and were trying to leave behind. Feminist scholar Arlene Voski Avakian was one of the few academics who highlighted the pleasures, as well as the tribulations, of cooking in her 1997 edited volume *Through the Kitchen Window: Women Explore the Intimate Meanings of Food and Cooking.*

As a woman a generation younger than these pioneering women academics, I did not feel the same tensions and constraints regarding domestic food production. On the contrary, I was intrigued by the topic. I began collecting articles and books that became very important in the development of my thinking, including works by historians Warren Belasco, Joan Jacobs Brumberg, Carolyn Bynum, Alfred Crosby, William Cronon, Carolyn Merchant, and Harvey Levenstein and anthropologists Claude Fischler, Sidney Mintz, Carole Counihan, and Mary J. Weismantel. In addition to pioneering new interdisciplinary work that featured food, my work was also shaped by national conversations and events including government policy such as the surgeon general's report and the early 1990s revision of the four food groups to the food guide pyramid (which I later learned was heavily shaped by Marion Nestle).

A few key works of cultural food history came out in the late 1980s and early 1990s that heavily influenced young scholars of my cohort. First, Sidney Mintz's *Sweetness and Power* (1985) was revelatory. A cultural history of the production and consumption of sugar, *Sweetness and*

Power was central to the development of food studies in general. Mintz, an anthropologist, extensively detailed and analyzed the transatlantic production and consumption of sugar from the colonial era through the mid-twentieth century, weaving into the story economics, colonization, industrialization, cultural meanings of sugar and their alteration over time, nutrition and health, and issues of class, labor, and race. Mintz deftly and inextricably linked the Caribbean enslaved, who planted, harvested, and processed the sugar, to the British working classes, who as the backbone of the Industrial Revolution consumed vast quantities of that sugar as a significant portion of their daily caloric intake. Further, Mintz made remarkable use of a wide variety of sources, including recipe books, a fact that made at least one reviewer regard the book with less legitimacy as a result of its using such "trivial" domestic sources (even though they were archived in the British Library) (Bentley 2008). Finally, Mintz's book was unique in that it put an edible commodity squarely at the center of the work and examined it from all angles, using multiple methods and theoretical frameworks. Although it was not unheard of to write about a specific food before *Sweetness and Power* (see, for example, Salaman 1949), Mintz's book legitimized the practice, and dozens of single-food histories have been published since.

Other influential works of cultural food history in the late 1980s featured food and gender more prominently, including Patricia Curran's *Grace before Meals: Food Ritual and Body Discipline in Convent Culture* (1989) and Joan Jacobs Brumberg's *Fasting Girls: The History of Anorexia Nervosa* (1988). Curran, a former nun, wrote an ethnography of meals, meal rituals, and approaches to food in two different convents. Included in her research were maps of the refectories where the nuns took their meals. She showed that the women's approach to food (more ascetic, more celebratory) depended on when they entered the convent, whether before or after Vatican II, a series of reforms that helped usher the church from the medieval period into the twentieth century. Brumberg's *Fasting Girls* also intertwined gender and food to understand young girls' lack of power and control and how this was manifested through eating, and avoiding, food. *Fasting Girls*, along with Caroline Walker Bynum's *Holy Fast, Holy Feast: The Religious Significance of Food to Medieval Women* (1988), explored similar themes. Also instrumental as models for food-focused cultural history was Warren Belasco's *Appetite for Change: How the Counterculture Took on the Food Industry* (1989). Belasco used his own experience as a 1960s college student and Boomer to write a history of the counterculture's effect on food. In these books, I discovered a model for the kind of research I sought to do: food-focused cultural history that drew upon other disciplines (psychology, nutrition, gender studies) for support and interpretation.

Further, a handful of fledgling institutions and organizations in the late 1980s helped provide academic and organizational structure for the study of culture, history, and food, most prominently the Association for the Study of Food and Society (ASFS). Begun in 1987, ASFS experienced the growing pains of a new field of study, but it confirmed that there was a critical mass of scholars drawn to food as a topic, including sociologists, historians, nutrition, early food activists, rural sociologists, and philosophers. The Agriculture, Food, and Human Values Society (AFHVS) was a similar organization founded at roughly the same time though more tilted toward sustainability and social justice issues.

The shape and makeup of NYU food studies (I joined the department in 1996) provided structure as I shaped my dissertation into a book manuscript, particularly by foregrounding issues of nutrition science and history. As academics trained in nutrition, department colleagues Marion Nestle and Sharron Dalton alerted me to the fact that I could not talk about vitamin-enriched bread prior to World War II, because it had only been enriched in the 1940s as part of the war effort. This eye-opening exchange and others like it helped me understand that nutrition had a history, a history I needed to reckon with in my work. Engagement with nutrition students and faculty led me to consider not just the historical and cultural but also the materiality of food, its nutritional and chemical properties. The latter, I realized, is so important when trying to understand, for example, cooking techniques and traditions. What does a "slow oven" mean in nineteenth-century cookbooks? How do coal and wood-fire ovens, as opposed to electric, gas, or microwave ovens, shape food, cuisine, and culture? What happens to food when cooked in a microwave, preventing any aromas from being emitted during cooking? How and why is it important to understand food making as craft and the impulse to cook and produce food by hand as a bulwark against anomie vis-à-vis industrialization? Further, this emerging science and technology as applied to food work fostered a distinctly gendered version known as "domestic science," which helped shaped ideas about food and nutrition for decades (Lears 1982; Sennett 2008; Shapiro 2008; Sutton 2014; Trubek 2017; Wallach 2019).

The structural and institutional constraints of NYU food studies fostered two guiding principles that informed my ongoing research: a cultural/historical framework enriched through nutrition/food as material perspectives (particularly my work on baby food); and the goal of writing scholarship that would appeal not only to academics of different stripes but to the larger public. As I look back at my body of work, I see a specific shaping of my research as a result of NYU food studies. In addition to my work on the history of baby food, my work on World War II and food rationing and my current project, a history of food in hospitals in the United States, are located within cultural food history and food studies, with distinct influence from nutritional sciences and nutrition history.

Indeed, my last book, *Inventing Baby Food: Taste, Health and the Industrialization of the American Diet* (2014) focuses on how ideas about health, the body, and infant food and feeding changed over the decades based on (among other things) the discovery of vitamins, the ramping up of canned goods, distribution networks, advertising, and also childrearing theories and even ideas about postwar national exceptionalism. It is mostly a historical work, but the last chapter does examine infant food and feeding trends in the 2010s (right up to publication). I have given dozens of talks over the years, and invariably the question most asked is, What is the best way to feed my baby? Not a historical question, but what to do now. I can and do answer these questions, but I also point out that women have asked these very same questions for a long time. The book explores the history of infant feeding advice, demonstrating that anxieties about infant feeding have always existed. It makes sense, as it is quite a felt responsibility to make sure one's baby survives and thrives. It also is a concrete example of how important questions about food are to people today, how the past and academic inquiry can have bearing on the present day, and how NYU food studies' intimacy with nutrition research and empirical scholarship has shaped my own.

The study of food and gender within NYU food studies continues to evolve in important, exciting directions in tandem with the evolution of academic and popular understandings of gender. Taking cues from queer studies, we teach and discuss research on, for example, food work in same-sex households, masculinities and food, and the queering of food (see for example Carrington 2013; Ehrhardt 2018; Parasecoli 2013). Students as well as faculty are engaged in these conversations, as highlighted by colleague Jennifer Berg's popular *Advanced Seminar on Food and Gender*.

It is impossible to predict the future beyond the COVID pandemic and accompanying societal disruption and reordering. One would never wish the trauma we have collectively experienced to continue, but we must capture the silver lining in the darker cloud of the moment. Just as social movements and upheavals in the past have led to societal changes with regard to gender and ethnicity/race, so too must we seize this moment to improve both society and our societal and pedagogical critique. We must ensure that the foment of physical trauma of the coronavirus, the ensuing social unrest, and public enlightenment over structural racism during the pandemic has shaped, and will continue to shape, NYU food studies and its broader environs.

REFERENCES

Avakian, Arlene Voski, ed. 1997. *Through the Kitchen Window: Women Explore the Intimate Meanings of Food and Cooking*. Boston: Beacon.

Belasco, Warren. 1989. *Appetite for Change: How the Counterculture Took on the Food Industry*. Ithaca, NY: Cornell University Press.

Bentley, Amy. 1998. *Eating for Victory: Food Rationing and the Politics of Domesticity*. Urbana: University of Illinois Press.

———. 2008. "Introduction" *Food and Foodways* 16 (2): 111–116.

———. 2012. "Sustenance, Abundance, and the Place of Food in United States Histories." In *Global Food Historiography: Researchers, Writers, & the Study of Food*, edited by Kyri Claflin and Peter Scholliers, 72–86. London: Bloomsbury.

———. 2014. *Inventing Baby Food: Taste, Health and the Industrialization of the Joan American Diet*. Oakland: University of California Press.

Brumberg, Joan Jacobs. 1988. *Fasting Girls: The History of Anorexia*. Ithaca, NY: Cornell University Press.

Bynum, Carolyn Walker. 1988. *Holy Feast, Holy Fast: The Religious Significance of Food to Medieval Women*. San Francisco: University of California Press.

Carrington, Christopher. 2013. "Feeding LesBiGay Families." In *Food and Culture: A Reader*, edited by Carole Counihan and Penny Van Esterik, 198–204. New York. Routledge.

Counihan, Carole. 1999. *The Anthropology of Food and the Body: Gender, Meaning, Power*. New York. Routledge.

Cronon, William. 1983. *Changes in the Land: Indians, Colonists, and the Ecology of New England*. New York: Hill and Wang.

Crosby, Alfred. 1973. *The Columbian Exchange: Biological and Cultural Consequences of 1492*. Westport, CT: Greenwood.

Dahlberg, Frances, ed. 2009. *Women the Gatherer*. New Haven, CT: Yale University Press.

Ehrhardt, Julia C. 2018. "Towards Queering Food Studies: Foodways, Heteronormativity, and Hungry Women in Chicana Lesbian Writing." In *Food and Culture: A Reader*, edited by Carole Counihan and Penny Van Esterik, 163–76. New York Routledge.

Fischler, Claude. 1990. *L'Homnivore: Sur les Fondamentaux de la Biologie et de la Philosophie*. Paris: Odile Jacob.

Gibbons, Ann. 2020. "Woman the Hunter, Ancient Andean Remains Challenge Old Ideas of Who Speared Big Game," *Science*, November 4. https://www.science.org.

Gussow, Joan. 1980. "Some Impractical Thoughts on Television & Nutritional Education." *Food Monitor* (November/December). Available at http://joansgarden.org/.

Haas, Randall, James Watson, Tammy Buonasera, John Southon, Jennifer C. Chen, Sarah Noe, Kevin Smith, et al. 2020. "Female Hunters of the Early Americas." *Science Advances* 6 (45). doi: 10.1126/sciadv.abd0310.

Harris, Marvin. 1998. *Good to Eat: Riddles of Food and Culture*. Long Grove, IL: Waveland.

Hedenstierna-Jonson, Charlotte, Anna Kjellström, Torun Zachrisson, Maja Krzewińska, Veronica Sobrado, Neil Price, Torsten Günther, et al. 2017. "A Female Viking Warrior Confirmed by Genetics," *American Journal of Physical Anthropology* 164 (4): 853–60. https://doi.org/10.1002/ajpa.23308

Kelly, Eleanor. 2012. "Knowing Our History and Culture Helps Us Build a Sense of Pride." *Open Society Foundation*, September 6. https://www.opensocietyfoundations.org.

Lears, T. J. Jackson. 1981. *No Place of Grace: Antimodernism and the Transformation of American Culture, 1880–1920*. New York: Pantheon.

Levenstein, Harvey. 1988. *Revolution at the Table: The Transformation of the American Diet*. Oxford: Oxford University Press.

Lévi-Strauss, Claude. 2008. "The Culinary Triangle," in *Food and Culture: A Reader*, edited by Carole Counihan and Penny Van Esterik, 21–28. New York. Routledge.

Mintz, Sidney 1985. *Sweetness and Power: The Place of Sugar in Modern History*. New York: Viking.

Merchant, Carolyn. 1989. *Ecological Revolutions: Nature, Gender, and Science in New England* Chapel Hill: University of North Carolina Press.

Newitz, Annalee. 2021. "What New Science Techniques Tell Us about Ancient Women Warriors. *New York Times*, January 1. www.newyorktimes.com.

Parasecoli, Fabio. 2013. "Feeding Hard Bodies: Food and Masculinities in Men's Fitness Magazines." In *Food and Culture: A Reader*, edited by Carole Counihan and Penny Van Esterik, 284–88. New York: Routledge.

Ray, Krishnendu. 2019. "ASFS Presidential Address: Towards an Epistemology of Pleasure and Post-Liberal Politics of Joy." *Food, Culture and Society* 22 (1): 3–8. doi: 10.1080/15528014.2018.1547068.

Richards, Audrey. 1939. *Land, Labour, and Diet in Northern Rhodesia: An Economic Study of the Bemba Tribe.* Oxford: Oxford University Press.

Salaman, Redcliffe. 1949. *The History and Social Influence of the Potato.* Cambridge, UK: Cambridge University Press.

Sennett, Richard. 2008. *The Craftsman.* New Haven, CT: Yale University Press.

Shapiro, Laura. 2008. *Perfection Salad: Women and Cooking at the Turn of the Century.* New York: Farrar, Strauss and Giroux.

Sutton, David E. 2014. *Secrets from the Greek Kitchen: Cooking, Skill, and Everyday Life on an Aegean Island.* Berkeley: University of California Press.

Trubek, Amy B. 2017. *Making Modern Meals: How Americans Cook Everyday.* Oakland: University of California Press.

Wallach, Jennifer Jensen. 2019. *Every Nation Has Its Dish: Black Bodies and Black Food in Twentieth Century America.* Chapel Hill: University of North Carolina Press.

Weismantel, Mary J. 1998. *Food, Gender and Poverty in the Ecuadorian Andes.* Waveland.

Welter, Barbara. 1966. "The Cult of True Womanhood." *American Quarterly* 18 (2): 151–74.

Wolf, Eric R. 1982. *Europe and the People without a History.* San Francisco: University of California Press.

Wrangham, Richard. 2010. *Catching Fire: How Cooking Made Us Human.* New York: Basic Books.

Yoder, Donald. 1972a. "Folk Cookery." In *Folklore and Folklife: An Introduction*, edited by Richard Dorson, 325–50. Chicago: University of Chicago Press.

———. 1972b. "Folk Costume." In *Folklore and Folklife: An Introduction*, edited by Richard Dorson, 295–324. Chicago: University of Chicago Press.

———. 1972c. "Folk Medicine." In *Folklore and Folklife: An Introduction*, edited by Richard Dorson, 191–216]]. Chicago: University of Chicago Press.

2

Sociology

Migrant Food Cultures

KRISHNENDU RAY

Coming to Food Studies

I came to Food Studies via an absence. I was ten thousand miles away from home in the United States, and I did not know how to cook to feed myself. In the process, I had to confront the fact that learning to cook had never even been a thought until my emigration. That void opened to me the power of an anthropological insight: that sometimes the most important aspect of a culture is hidden in plain view, taken for granted, until an outsider shows up with a different habitus. In my case, the ethnographic act was to enter a new social-cultural order of another nation-state, which then lit up what was invisible to me before leaving. Immigration in itself provided an epistemological opening. In that sense I see myself as an inverted anthropologist.

This quotidian aspect of life—cooking, eating, serving, and sharing— opened up a vast sphere of the un-thought-through for me. I began to fill my ignorance with a curious collection of books. In the early 1990s, there weren't that many books explicitly and exclusively on food culture, especially cooked food in domestic settings. There were, however, lots of books and tons of literature on hunger, political-economy of hunger and the Green Revolution, and the international food system and inequality. I was familiar with Amartya Sen's work on hunger and entitlement and Norman Borlaug's and M. S. Swaminathan's research on the Green Revolution. As a teenager, I had participated fully in the technocratic national propaganda on the coming utopia of hybrid wheat, fertilizer, and irrigation. I was also familiar with Gandhi's spectacular fasts as techniques of political mobilization. I was somewhat familiar with cookbooks but ignored them as trivial ephemera.

This was likely the product of my undergraduate training in political-economy and political science. I learned later that those productivist concerns had been primarily contained in the domain of political-economy since the physiocrats. The gap between my knowledge and my self-awareness was in the realm of everyday consumption; that was yet to emerge as a new field of inquiry. I was hungry for some analysis of a cooking, eating, caring subject and of its social production. Where could I find analysis of the cooking and eating practices of modern, urban, mobile subjects like myself?

That is when I stumbled sequentially—since there was no defined discipline or even a well-defined inter-disciplinary intersection that could systematically bound my query—into a number of trajectory-defining books. In the home of my professor, Giovanni Arrighi, I learned to eat my first pizza and stomach grappa along with an array of other Third World graduate students from Namibia, Egypt, Chile, Pakistan, and Afghanistan. Arrighi, an early scholar of global capitalism and an erudite teacher, and his partner, Beverly Silver, the famous sociologist of labor, gave us a safe harbor and unimaginable things to eat at their home in the dying white working-class town of Binghamton. It was also where I caught sight of a copy of Jack Goody's *Cooking, Cuisine and Class*. Goody's book was a massive comparative thesis on the relations between technologies of production, writing, and hierarchy of taste, and the resultant difference in cuisines and in culture between Sub-Saharan Africa and Eurasia—the perfect book to stumble upon, given the global context of my newly acquired friends and neighbors.

Subsequently, I learned about the writings of Mary Douglas on everyday meals in a British middle-class home and Claude Lévi-Strauss's excruciatingly detailed Gallic theorization on the raw, the cooked, and the rotten. I still remember the thrill of finding scholars describing and theorizing changing patterns of food consumption, such as Pierre Bourdieu, who would subsequently come to dominate the field of cultural sociology. Quickly that led back to the semiotic work of Roland Barthes, the social history of Fernand Braudel in his three volumes of *Civilization and Capitalism*, and finally back again to the political-economy of Sidney Mintz's *Sweetness and Power*, which was both material and symbolic. In the process of familiarizing myself with the emerging an-thropology, sociology, and history of consumption and reproduction, I also stumbled into Laura Shapiro's *Perfection Salad*—a study of the Boston Cooking School at the end of nineteenth century—and Harvey Levenstein's *Paradox of Plenty*. They reoriented me to food culture in the context of overabundant consumerism, new to me given my origins in the context of scarcity, where even middle-class children suffer from malnutrition and are often stunted and wasted. The paradox of having too much food of poor quality was a new problem that I had to reorient myself to.

All this reading and thinking, cooking and cleaning, done abroad, was changing my mind. I went to my advisor and said, "Mark, I would like to change my dissertation from questions of development and un-derdevelopment to questions of migration and changes in everyday life, specifically food preparation and consumption." He tried to talk me out of it. I was fixated, as I tend to be, on my new questions, without overt considerations of career. But I had softened him enough that when he ran across an advertisement in the *Chronicle of Higher Education* for a position to develop a curriculum on the history and cultures of Asia and the Americas at the Culinary Institute of America (CIA), he passed it on to me and encouraged me to apply. I never thought I would get the job, because I did not know anything about Western haute cuisine and had not even had a glass of wine. But I was excited. As I later learned, CIA's leadership had come to recognize that to produce leaders in the culinary profession, they had to train students not only to be exemplary cooks, bakers, and sommeliers but also to be concerned about developing a point of view on sustainability, wellness, and cultural difference. They were astute at identifying three things that would drive the dynamics of the emergent urban American public culture of food. This was in the mid-1990s, and there was a lot of excitement in the professional world of chefs, commentators, critics, and television programmers about the quickly expanding world that exceeded the old concerns around stuffy old gourmandise and narrow interests of an occupational guild.

Food Network, for instance, was being reorganized by Erica Gruen in 1996 to move away from talking-head shows for those who loved to cook to more action-packed programming for consumers—those who liked to eat—that made the network ubiquitous in almost every

American household. My students at the CIA were the most excited by a weird, campy, Japanese program called *Iron Chef*. It was structured as an intense competition between Japanese chefs with dubbed commentary. Often quaint and exotic, with interesting ingredients such as octopus and shark or mushrooms, the programs were focused on craft, ingredients, and skills of cooking and evaluating quality. My students, mostly white working-class men with a sprinkling of wayward children of white and Asian professionals, were excited both about the possibility of knowledge and respect for ingredients and profession and about the campy, ironic, not to be taken too seriously voice-over of the program.

In retrospect, it is surprising how important that TV program was. The extension of a Japanese cultural sensibility about forms of craft masculinity, conveyed through an entertaining TV program, was an early hint of the reorientation of global public culture toward East Asian imports from Japan, Taiwan, and Korea that we are still living through. *Iron Chef* was so successful that it would morph into its own American version and one of the sources of a new emerging public American conversation about food. Marshall McLuhan (1964, 54) had already predicted that TV would be more hospitable to a tactile visual skillset such as cooking and would appeal to performers who did not need high-cultural skills of reading and writing. Literary ballast to this pop sensibility would be provided a little later by Anthony Bourdain's *Kitchen Confidential*, published in 2000. *Iron Chef* and *Kitchen Confidential* quickly became two touchstones of the most engaged discussions among students at the CIA around craft, class, gender, and cultural difference in thinking, writing, and doing food. Two contextual referents are important here: that I was teaching at a culinary school and outside an established discipline allowed me the room to pay attention to what could have been dismissed as too popular for a scholar. Disciplines discipline their practitioners by excluding distracting material from our attention. Sometimes they exclude emergent data from analysis. That would be one of the spaces of emergence of food studies.

Another issue that had been percolating, first as a countercultural sensibility on sustainability, gurgling on the margins since *Silent Spring* and *A Diet for a Small Planet*, was Alice Water's offensive against the sedate industrial norms of the profession of hotel cooking. To my boisterous students, if Masaharu Morimoto and Anthony Bourdain were surefire heroes in the domain of craft and culture, the more thoughtful and better-read ones took up the cudgels for Waters's seasonal, sustainable restaurant, Chez Panisse. It was the calling card of a small band of feminists, vegetarians, critical theorists, artists and all-around bookworms who had somehow ended up at the CIA, which was otherwise a militaristic male organization. It is worth noting that this analytical frame for understanding the ecological crisis and the problems engendered by the agro-industrial food system was also transforming NYU's Home Economics department into the current iteration of Nutrition and Food Studies under the leadership of Marion Nestle, who by her own account would be nudged toward food studies by a California restaurant consultant, Clark Wolf. Those countercultural but profession-making impulses were driven by the younger teachers and chefs at the CIA, and their perspectives on locality and seasonality were often fed by their experiences with California cuisine in the Napa Valley.

That would be the entry point of a major transformation in the culture of instructor chefs, who until then were quite comfortable with mass produced industrial foods and often built their careers first in the agro-industrial food complex. They would incorporate the Chez Panisse perspective as a critique in the name of flavor and sustainability. Yet the dominant culture of old Euro-American five-star hotel chefs would not concede ground easily. That fight would be fought out between the older and the younger chefs. The conflict simmered for almost two decades between 1975 and 1995 at the CIA. By the twenty-first century, what had been dominant—careers in the industrial food sector—would still remain the unspoken presumption, yet high-end restaurants with the chef as the craftsman if not artiste, attentive to farmers' markets and the work of local farmers and butchers, would emerge as the new and highly visible protagonists in the food system. If food TV provided examples of alternative cultural idioms from the Pacific region, California cuisine provided another frame to understand and argue for ecological sustainability and care of the earth, bodies, and communities of production and consumption. These two emerging points of view crystallized into the new American perspective on sustainability, human and animal health, and cultural difference, the very things leaders of the CIA, Ferdinand Metz and Tim Ryan, had begun to articulate when they hired me to work on the liberal arts curriculum at a professional school.

In the Nutrition and Food Studies Department at NYU, where I now teach, students collect in three clusters: one in the area of policy and advocacy, another in the domain of social entrepreneurship, and finally in the sphere of culture and communication. The foundational class I teach, Contemporary Issues in Food Studies, covers about a dozen topics. The goal is to get students coming from diverse disciplines, undergraduate majors, and professional experience on the same page and introduce them to quantitative and qualitative research and provide them with a vocabulary to sort information within a conceptual framework. We are in the strictest sense a multidisciplinary program teaching our students the content and techniques from various disciplines, from quantitative social sciences, survey data collection, and ethnographic work to archival work in the humanities, including performance studies. If there is one thing they learn in that course, it is how to think and write as a producer of knowledge rather than as a mere consumer. The topics range from political ecology, gender and care work, urban infrastructure, immigrants in the food system, sensory evaluation, and aesthetic theory to eating animals, cellular agriculture, and waste. In each subsequent semester, they dig deeper into a domain and acquire greater depth in lieu of the breadth of their first two semesters and are taught by experts in history, cultural studies, media studies, economics, photography, digital humanities, and policy making. My job is to prime students to accommodate vast amounts of data and complex evidence-based studies within a framework of concepts and express their considered judgment about those issues in clear-cut output, in words, and/or in numbers.

My research, girded by the qualitative social sciences and the humanities, informs my teaching that food culture is not only about culinary roots but also about the routes of dispersal of people, plants, and animals. *The Migrant's Table* (2004), my first book based on surveys of 126 immigrant households, showed how food matters to respondents' conceptions of self and the other and how the migrant body, in crossing national boundaries, could become a tool equal to the anthropological device of the informed outsider. My second book, *Curried Cultures* (2012) (co-edited with Tulasi Srinivas), explored globalization and South Asia from the colonial period to the postcolonial era as seen through the aperture of the senses. My third book, *The Ethnic Restaurateur* (2016), showed that immigrants from many parts of the world—Irish, German,

Chinese, Indian, Mexican, among others—have been central to feeding occupations in the United States since data on birthplace and occupations has been collected, beginning with the 1850 census. Out of that empirical work, I developed an argument about the historical process of profession-making in the matrix of class, race, gender, and ethnicity that I will detail below.

Hierarchy of Taste

There I developed the concept of a hierarchy of taste—after Jack Goody and Michael Herzfeld—regarding the relationship between demographics, popularity, and prestige of cuisines. For instance, only 2 percent of Indian restaurants in New York City were upscale in 2019, while 12 percent of Italian restaurants and 27 percent of French restaurants were so. On the other hand, Italian, Chinese, and Mexican restaurants were the most popular, although very few restaurants among the last two categories could break into the domain of pricey prestige. That distribution of popularity and hierarchy is currently different in London, for instance, where both Italian and Indian are popular and can be prestigious. That concept and the data it is based on has dramatically shaped the public discussion of restaurant reviewing in the United States (Carmen 2018).

The robust public discussion of my (largely academic) book included a piece in the *Atlantic*, which published a multi-page issue on it with a number of figures along with an interview titled "The Future Is Expensive Chinese Food," which drew on my analysis of the past to project into the future (Pinsker 2016). Both the *Atlantic* and the *Washington Post* included data visualization from my book (reproduced below) (Ferdman 2016; Ramanathan 2015). In that work, I ranked cuisines by average price in the New York City market over thirty years. Check averages show a clear hierarchy of taste: French, American (especially New American), and continental lead the pack in terms of prestige. Italian follows closely; most notably, Japanese restaurants have leapfrogged to the top rank from number five in terms of price. The fastest climbing ones are Japanese, Greek, and Korean, with some signs of upward mobility for Vietnamese and marginally Mexican cuisines in the Zagat dataset. As I have shown elsewhere, the Yelp dataset shows some similarities and

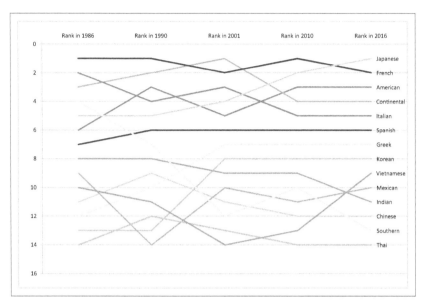

Figure 2.1: Rank of Zagat average price of a meal by self-identified category of restaurant, select years (1986—first available; 1990, 2001, 2010, 2016 latest price data available). Graph by Krishnendu Ray.

differences. *Los Angeles Times*' restaurant critic Patricia Escárcega put it succinctly: "It's getting better, but food journalism still has a pervasive race and class problem" (Peterson 2019). The reason is that while cooking, cleaning, and serving are working-class occupations, fine dining is dominated by the demands of the rich. In that context, I came to describe *ethnic food*—food of the poor, recent immigrants of color—as the shattered mirror of haute cuisine. Both the data and the *data visualization* has been central to making the argument succinctly and persuasively leading to its wide dissemination.

This is to illustrate that the field of food studies, specifically my research on immigrants and American foodways, is informing the wider public discussion on culture, power, and social structure (Wang 2016). This is important because the basic division in American politics is the gulf between the highly educated and the less formally educated, which is driving much of the right-wing revanchist populism. My attempt is to bridge that space, connecting work inside the academy to the world outside. Similarly, I, along with a dozen other colleagues, are trying to do the same in driving *Gastronomica*, a food studies journal, toward greater public engagement via podcasts and better visual materials and in paying as much attention to creative as to critical scholarly work. As a result of that public engagement, my broader thinking on the future of the immigrant-dominated restaurant industry after COVID-19 has begun to shape editorials in the *Los Angeles Times* and *Eater* (Peterson 2021; Zhang 2020). There I argue that some of the cost of a restaurant meal has to be internalized in the price of a product, some of it socialized via mechanisms such as universal health care, and some of it shared as cooperative costs such as the development of less predatory delivery apps.

My next book, *The Death of the Street Vendor*, investigates the structural role played by state regulation, city planning, and corporate supermarkets in the making and unmaking of street vending and marketplaces. What has been lost and what has been gained in that process? Who has won and who has lost in the proliferation of the supermarket system of provisioning? In it, I analyze rural-to-urban migration and the built environment of food provisioning, urban infrastructure, and social media networks in the Global North and the Global South. Urban provisioning in India is on the cusp of the changes already completed in places such as the United States. My analysis opens with the impact of COVID-19 on small markets but interrogates deeper and longer processes of provisioning and supply-chain making. It looks closely at the intended and unintended consequences of provisioning in the model of supermarkets, suburbia, and automobility, which has been the product of a constellation of forces unleashed by the American century. Although fewer than one billion people own cars in the world today, they dramatically shape the lives of the other seven billion, including how they feed themselves. That American century, with its model of urban provisioning, is coming to an end now, revealing the costs in terms of inequality, the health of the population and the environment, and urban planning. This is also an attempt to shift away from the overbearing Euro-American provincialism that has dominated food studies since its birth in the Global North. This book will be the final volume of my trilogy on mobility, materiality, and migrant food culture.

In Closing

I have engaged most intensely with journalists and advocates rather than sociologists in my career. That is not the standard way of going about the business of doing research. Usually, people come to a field in graduate school with their interest and affective investments, and shoehorn them into current discussions in a discipline. If that were my practice I would have to stick to the sociology of immigration or the sociology of consumption or the sociology of inequality—primarily because my PhD was in sociology—and probably I would have touched on food and then moved on to other things to illustrate disciplinary concerns. In fact, too much attention to a thing such as food could be a career killer in any discipline, even today. That is linked to the peculiar history of the making of disciplines in American universities at the end of the nineteenth century—modeled after the German research university—when cooked food fell off the plate as a legitimate domain of expert knowledge (Geiger 1986, 1993; Grendler 2002; Lawrence 1974; Ross 1990; Rueschemeyer and Skocpol 2017).

Instead of a discipline, I inhabit an intersection called food studies, where food is the anchoring object. In addition, I am an immigrant of color. That shapes my experience and my conceptions, as much as analogous locations were instigations for the great theorists of sociology. So location matters, and institutional ecology matters. My work, at the broadest level, can be characterized as the study of subject-object relations in the light of new materialisms and affect theory. The secret is to find a productive niche, as much in the social world as in the natural world. I draw on sociological subdomains—immigration, valuation, inequality, consumption—but I stay away from subdisciplinary contestation. My orientation is not primarily to other sociologists but to my students and a broader public, which is quintessentially a food studies location. That shapes my methods and language of description and analysis. All knowledge exists in networks, and those are some of mine. Second, I borrow methods, content, and topic equally from a number of adjacent disciplines, especially history, anthropology, cultural studies, and folklore, which makes me less anchored in disciplinary discussions. I find the intersections between them rather than the boundaries among them. The latter is central to discipline making and the most important imperative to new scholars in the field. To get a job and keep one, they need to underline the virtues of their discipline over others. I was lucky to escape that imperative because I skirted the boundaries of a number of them from the very beginning when I started teaching at a cooking school. I began with immigrant foodways, moved to the adjacent domain of immigrant entrepreneurship, and am now moving to micro-entrepreneurship of the poor in the Global South. At every turn, I have been pushed by the nature and limits of my experience and history, by my own curiosity, and by the public that I have crafted over the last two decades.

REFERENCES

Bourdain, Anthony. 2000. *Kitchen Confidential*. New York: Bloomsbury.

Braudel, Fernand. 1992. *Civilization and Capitalism. Vol. 1–3*. Berkeley: University of California Press.

Carmen, Tim. 2018. "My Column's Name Does a Disservice to the Immigrants Whose Food I Celebrate So I'm Dropping It." *Washington Post*, December 31. https://www.washingtonpost.com.

Carson, Rachel. 1962. *Silent Spring*. Houghton Mifflin.

Dickie, George. 1996. *The Century of Taste*. New York: Oxford University Press.

Ferdman, Roberto A. 2016. "How Americans Pretend to Love 'Ethnic Food.'" *Washington Post*, April 22. https://www.washingtonpost.com.

Geiger, Roger L. 1986. *To Advance Knowledge*. New York: Oxford University Press.

———. 1993. *Research and Relevant Knowledge: American Research Universities since World War II*. New York: Oxford University Press.

Goody, Jack. 1996. *Cooking, Cuisine and Class*. Cambridge, UK: Cambridge University Press.

Grendler, Paul F. 2002. *The Universities of the Italian Renaissance*. Baltimore, MD: Johns Hopkins University Press.

Herzfeld, Michael. 2003. *The Body Impolitic. Artisans and Artifice in the Global Hierarchy of Value*. Chicago: University of Chicago Press.

Korsmeyer, Carolyn. 1999. *Making Sense of Taste*. Ithaca, NY: Cornell University Press.

Lappé, Francis Moore. 1991. *Diet for a Small Planet*. New York: Ballantine.

Levenstein, Harvey. 2003. *Paradox of Plenty: A Social History of Eating in Modern America*. Berkeley: University of California Press.

McLuhan, Marshall. 1964. *Understanding Media: The Extensions of Man*. New York: Signet.

Mintz, Sidney. 1986. *Sweetness and Power*. New York: Penguin.

Peterson, Lucas Kwan. 2019. "Q&A: Get to Know Patricia Escárcega, New Restaurant Critic for The L.A. Times." *Los Angeles Times*, January 10. https://www.latimes.com.

———. 2021. "We Should Pay More to Eat in Restaurants." *Los Angeles Times*, March 19. https://www.latimes.com.

Pinsker, Joe. 2016. "The Future Is Expensive Chinese Food." *Atlantic*, July 13. https://www.theatlantic.com.

Ramanthan, Lavanya. 2015. "Why Everyone Should Stop Calling Immigrant Food 'Ethnic.'" *Washington Post*, July 21. https://www.washingtonpost.com.

Ray, Krishnendu. 2004. *The Migrant's Table*. Philadelphia: Temple University Press.

———. 2016. *The Ethnic Restaurateur*. London: Bloomsbury.

Ray, Krishnendu, and Tulasi Srinivas, eds. 2014. *Curried Cultures*. Berkeley: University of California Press.

Ross, Dorothy. 1990. *The Origins of American Social Science*. Cambridge, UK: Cambridge University Press.

Rueschemeyer, Dietrich, and Theda Skocpol, eds. 2017. *States, Social Knowledge, and the Origins of Modern Social Policies*. Princeton, NJ: Princeton University Press.

Shapiro, Laura. 1986. *Perfection Salad*. New York: Farrar, Straus & Giroux.

Stone, Lawrence. 1974. *The University in Society*. 2 vols. Princeton, NJ: Princeton University Press.

Wang, Esther. 2016. "New Wave of Chinese Restaurants Challenges 'Cheap' Stereotype." *NPR, The Salt*, November 14. https://www.npr.org.

Zhang, Jenny G. 2020. "The Future of Restaurants Depends on Universal Healthcare." *Eater*, September 1. https://www.eater.com.

3

Poetry and Literary Studies

Re/De/Composition of Food Studies

ERIC HIMMELFARB

On the first day of class, we begin with a discussion about Romanesco broccoli. Before introductions, before going over the syllabus, this is our entry point into a new semester of studying the poetics of food justice protest. A picture is projected on the screen and a question posed to the class: "What is the name of this beautiful, psychedelic piece of produce you see here, and what makes it so special?" A few chuckles, a few moments of uncomfortable quiet and shifting in seats, and then maybe I offer up a clue. "If we have any math experts in here," I say, "then you might know this." It's a course called Food in the Arts: The Poetic Voice, so the odds of math majors being present are low, but you never know. Then a potentially more helpful hint: "If you know something about the patterns embedded in snowflakes or river deltas then you might know about this as well." Eventually, our answer emerges, with the name of the broccoli and the venture of a hesitant, not-quite-certain guess: "That's a fractal, isn't it?"

I am not a mathematician, but I am a poet. I have an affinity for things poetic in form, and I can see that the Romanesco broccoli is nothing if not poetic. The brilliant lime green color is one thing, the taste is another, but it is the enchanting fractal formal essence of the broccoli that resonates most with me, as it eventually does with the students as well. For the other non-math people reading this and wondering what a fractal is: fractals "contain self-similar patterns of complexity increasing with magnification. If you divide a fractal pattern into parts you get a nearly identical reduced-size copy of the whole" (McNally 2010). Take another look at the Romanesco broccoli. Do you see the endlessly repeating patterns now? The way that the spiral at the level of the whole replicates itself at the level of the floret and on and on as you zoom in?

Romanesco broccoli consists of spirals of florets that themselves consist of spirals of florets. For the math experts who do happen to be reading this, this awe and amazement I'm expressing constitutes the full extent of my knowledge on this topic; consider it a fractal-for-poetry's-sake, nothing more and nothing less, and a fitting entry point both on this page and in the classroom.

Why would a poetry course in the NYU Nutrition and Food Studies Department begin this way? Right at the outset, a discussion about this concept sets the tone for the type of inquiry and creative imagining the course will encourage, as it invites the students to see food differently and to engage with it as a subject in an alternative way. Poetry has the ability to bring about these shifts in vision, and the class in general aims to do that as well. We look at poetry about food issues as an object of study, on the one hand, but on the other hand, we also approach poetry and poetic language as a method for conveying meaning about food and therefore as a method for reading, writing, and thinking about issues across the food system. So although the class certainly focuses on the art of poetry, we can also position this exploration as one that applies that art form, and that way of shaping language, to a particular set of social and environmental issues. The class—and my work more generally, by extension—thus emphasizes active storytelling, activism, and advocacy over observation and critique. We are all implicated in the joy of food, in the creative, generative aspects of the food system, as we are all implicated in the suffering and struggle, the destructive aspects of the same system. To engage in this nuanced space through the study and the writing of poetry means entering into the discussion in an active way.

Aside from setting the tone for the intended discourse of the semester, the fractal idea of a cyclical pattern that continuously reproduces itself at any and all levels of magnitude sets a thematic tone as well. We can see cyclical patterns made manifest within the food system across spatial and temporal bounds, particularly through or related to poetic expression. First, there are patterns at the level of *process*: the transformation of seed into crop is not that different from that of word into poem. Michael Pollan brings poetry and this type of natural transformation together while also building off Coleridge's theory of poetic creativity when he says that "fermentation is the secondary imagination of nature" (Pollan 2013, 404). In poetic composition, Pollan sees a parallel to the process of yeasts breaking down sugars: "Secondary imagination breaks down the substrate of ordinary experience . . . to create something . . . metaphorical: the strong wine of poetry where before there was only the ordinary juice of prose" (404). The pattern reproduces at any magnification, whether wine or poetry emerges.

The process of decomposed matter renewing itself into recomposed fertility in the form of compost and eventually new growth does not differ all that much from the way the composition of poetry takes the "sedimented" language of prose (King 2019, 2; Scigaj 1999, 13), deadened by commerce and politics and day-to-day mundanity, and elevates it into a new, recomposed form of the poem. Through a creative process of transformation, both mystical and mechanical, one form shifts into another and then appears to be a unified whole. The chaff of language is separated from the poetic grain, but the chaff of course finds use and life as recycled and recomposed matter elsewhere. In the way that a crop is not quite a finished product or an endpoint but is simply one stop in a cycle of growth, decay, and renewal, so too is a poem just one stop in a cyclical movement; ideas find form in words, words find new shapes and resonances, and they form new ideas in turn. In this sense, a poem continuously unfolds, never quite complete; it finds composition but also de- and recomposition through revisions and readings and new takes on universal themes that poets have grappled with since the beginning of poetry. When I read an old poem now, and it spurs me to action or even just spurs new visions in my mind, the poem has entered the current moment as in a constellation of forces that act in ways both tangible and intangible. In this manner, a poem actively recomposes itself; it does not just sit encased in glass in a museum, frozen in time and inert. Poems are "interbeings," as Maureen McLane terms them when speaking specifically about the ballad form. They are always in process and in progress toward another poem or form, never quite settled (McLane 2017, 112). In this unsettled state, poems provide a staging ground for the de- and recomposition of complexity: "I make my poems to make a way through what I often perceive as mess. . . . If my writing makes a mess of things, it's not to flee understanding but to map (mis-)understanding as a verb" (Kearney 2015, 29).

Then there are patterns on the level of *product*; zoom all the way out, and we can see it in full form from a distance like the Romanesco broccoli—the recurring concerns, from our earliest poets to current ones, about land stewardship, about environmental and food justice, about a spiritual, communal connection to the food we share and the land that provides it. We can see the admonitions, prophetic in tone, about how to grapple with our inescapable fragility and precariousness (since the written poetry we have is less than half as old as agriculture itself, worries about going hungry or facing a failing crop are not new), and we see expressions of doubt as to how much control we really can exert in our partnership with the ecological processes on which we rely in order to eat. Zoom back in to the level of a single poem itself, like a single floret, and we see how these expansive ideas, which seem to stretch from one end of the earth to the other, find their particular form in specific language on the page.

Through my earlier studies of English literature and poetry, through urban farm work, to graduate work in food studies and professional on-the-ground anti-hunger work in New York City, I have arrived at this synthesis as the core of my explorations as a scholar; I seek to understand the architecture of these patterns within food-related poetry—its key threads, the way it shapes language into form to express those threads, and its relevance and resonance for us in our current moment of ecological crises and social injustices across the food system. When poetry impacts us and sparks an idea about interconnectedness, how in fact does it do that? What brings about that resonance? My interest in this work has a lot to do with the writing of poetry in addition to the reading of it, since to compose poetry about food justice means to actively enter into that spiraling poetic fractal pattern across space and time of humans grappling with how to exist here together and sustain ourselves together and create meaning around that sustenance. The process (the composition and de- and recomposition) is as crucial as the end product (the poem, the crop, the fruit, the meal), and the process is, in a sense, the method of teaching the topic of food studies. My exploration, therefore, takes place along the marginal territory between critical work and creative output, between teaching and writing and researching, between directing an eye toward the poetic strategies and production of the past and toward crafting new ones, all in the hopes of constructing a blueprint of a poetry that might help to articulate the challenges we face in the food system, its inherent fragility on multiple planes and ways to imagine an alternative structure in increasingly perilous times.

This research must begin with a deceptively complicated set of questions: What does poetry do? What purposes does it truly serve, aside from aesthetic enjoyment? There can be a tension between theory and practice when studying food, in part because it forms the basis of our primal needs while still connecting to esoteric, political, and cultural aspects of our lives as well. But the method of studying food through poetry and the poetic mindset collapses some of that tension; poetry can be esoteric, and a poem can feel removed and abstract and inscrutable, yet at the same time, the poem has the potential to act in the world, through the creation of new vision. One answer to the question of what poetry does is that it *transforms*—language from sedimented into elevated, ideas into words and then new ideas in turn, conventional wisdom and ways of seeing the world into new ways. It can propel us toward concrete change, as it "forms the quality of light within which we predicate our hopes and dreams toward survival and change, first made into language, then into idea, then into more tangible action" (Lorde 1984, 37). Another answer is that poetry *connects*; through metaphor and simile, it brings together ideas, images, things, living beings and shows relations and interconnectedness where we may not have seen them before. And it makes what had been invisible more visible through novel language. It inspires in readers and writers, amid "the disorderly welter of subjectivity and imagination, the seeing and touching of another, of others, through language" (Rich 2003, xvi). Yet another answer is that it *enlivens* language that has become deadened or sedimented and in doing so shifts perception and vision as a "revelatory distillation of experience" (Lorde 1984, 37).

These core functions of poetry figure prominently when applied to the topic of the food system, since much of what ails that system can be linked back to structural disconnections inherent in the system—between producers and consumers, between laborers and eaters, between production methods and their environmental impacts, between those who are food secure and those who struggle to access adequate food. In a sense, the synthesis of this topic of study with this method of critical and creative inquiry serves as a response to various calls to action. In part, these calls range from the fact that 14.5 percent of global carbon emissions come from livestock production (FAO n.d.) and the other ways in which food production and consumption impact climate change, to the fact that 10.2 percent of Americans face food insecurity (USDA n.d.), and to the imperative to work for food sovereignty and food justice in this and other countries. At times, these pressing problems can feel remote and abstract. In enacting a sort of "slow violence," as Rob Nixon posits, these complex problems sometimes seem to occur gradually and out of sight, making a sense of urgency—not to mention an adequate representation in words or art—difficult to attain (Nixon 2011). My work takes these challenges, enveloped as we are in this era in certain intractable problems and complex issues, as a call to map out a new poetics around food and sustenance. The tools of metaphor and simile, among many others, provide the structural mechanisms for enacting these poetics and for connecting what before had seemed to be disconnected. This mapping may not equate directly or immediately to tangible policy change or to healthier soil (and this represents one of the fundamental tensions of this work), but the mapping itself brings forth imaginative elements that can and do impact the world.

We can hear calls to and for action in creative forms of representation. Fred Kirschenmann calls for "discovering a new mythology that will enable us to abandon the inventory-taking approach to agriculture" (Kirschenmann 2010, 270) that sees all natural resources as inventory to extract and exploit without worry for return or cycling back fertility, while Robin Wall Kimmerer writes of the need to compose a "new *ilbal*," a Mayan concept used to describe sacred stories, which she defines as "a precious seeing instrument, or lens, with which to view our sacred relationships" (Kimmerer 2013, 344). Poetry provides us with a mode, a technology, both new and ancient, for manifesting these alternative kinds of vision. Crucially, poetry, as both a form and a method, can help enact expansive connections, cyclical movements, and meaning-making maneuvers that might lead to a new mythology, or new lenses, to bring us closer to truly knowing, seeing, and understanding the subterranean and the cyclical in myriad facets and forms.

The word *poetry* derives from the Greek *poiesis*, which translates to "making." In writing poetry and dedicating that writing to the expansion of vision around food issues, we can, through words, make a new way of inhabiting our bodies and world. *Poiesis* "constitutes the breadth of aliveness rather than inaugurating the denigration of breath" (Quashie 2021, 46) and thus resides in the cyclical churn of soil organic matter and practices of daily survival as well as poetic practices and forms. While the disciplines of food studies and poetry are not obvious partners, food and poetry do in fact form a natural partnership through this generative act of *poiesis*. They feed and sustain us in different but necessary ways, and they speak to what makes us human and what brings us together with other humans and with the more-than-human.

Poetry about food is as old as poetry itself, and, perhaps more important, poetry about *fragility*—ecological, social, existential—is as old as poetry itself as well. Amitav Ghosh writes about the fact that "poetry . . . has long had an intimate relationship with climactic events" (Ghosh 2016, 26) and that "an awareness of the precariousness of human existence is to be found in every culture" (55), particularly in their ancient epic poetic texts. We should define fragility broadly here as it applies to the food system and note that not only does fragility relate to various ecological impacts and the realities of a changing climate that make agricultural conditions more difficult, but it also relates to the unsustainable human impacts of the food system, whether on laborers working on farms or in packing houses, on people around the world struggling to access food or not fully in control of their food production or policy. A system with such dire human impacts cannot be said to be sturdy and stable, suitable or sustainable.

How, in response to these calls to action, might poetry express, embody, and enact that sort of fragility in the food system? In this embodiment resides the seeds of change in the system—first of perception and later of more tangible markers. One exercise, toward the end of the semester, articulates an answer. With a couple of weeks remaining, we spend time writing poems on paper embedded with seeds, with instructions to the students to attempt planting their poems once they finish writing. We aim to write invocations—expressions of our fragility, recognitions that when we plant a seed we relinquish a good portion of control over what happens from there. Invocations may not mean much in the absence of regenerative soil-building techniques and other sound planting practices, but they certainly represent a method of putting into words what we find to be important and how we see ourselves fitting into the bigger picture. They remind us to feel and express gratitude and to maintain focus on what it will take for a good crop this year and next year and beyond, whatever that crop may be. Invocations written on seed paper, moreover, embody that fragility quite literally by establishing a tangible connection between words and seeds, between poetry and food. Through this exercise, then, we circle back to the idea of the fractal, as we begin to see the ways in which planting is like poetry and poetry is like planting. The crop will not emerge overnight, and neither will the poem. But we put our words underground, and we check back later to see what has emerged.

Another way to engage with the question of the poetic embodiment of fragility is to pose a different question—building off a continued study of the fractal poetic examples of the past—about what poetic composition should entail moving forward in this era of climate catastrophe, drought, wildfire, rising sea levels, and all the preexisting social strains they will exacerbate. This question, in tandem with the question of how to apply this to food system inequities in particular, forms the core of where this research will go from here. Ross Gay offers a preliminary answer when he writes, in "Catalog of Unabashed Gratitude," that "we built an orchard this way" (Gay 2015). Through the poem, he articulates this to mean: we built a community orchard through collaborative labor, by transporting compost and spent grains in wheelbarrows, propelled by the vision of courageous ancestors and of what it would mean to harvest fruit together years into the future. There is a poetics to this line, an architecture of meaning crafted through collectivity, creative vision, and the materiality of sustenance through food, and there is a politics, a call for a commons. We should thus aim for our response to be a cocreative process, a mode of creative critique, since we are collectively implicated in the food system, its impacts, and its potential repairs. McLane emphasizes the collaborative nature of poetry, saying that "poems, like people, thoughts, plants, and ballads themselves, are co-composed, are made and unmade together in a contingent networking of the animate and inanimate" (McLane 2017, 112). In this sense, a poem constitutes an "assemblage," a contingent co-composition, analogous to the broad "constellation of material things and social forces entangled in" food production (Guthman 2019, 25), for instance. The field of ecopoetics theorizes and extends this collaborative ethos, deploying "lyric ecologies" as a framework for analyzing methods of poetic composition and for modeling harmonious social and ecological relations (Posmentier 2017) and interrogating areas of alignment, resistance, skillful survival, and connectivity between humans and the natural world (Dungy 2009).

Our poems on seed paper in part reflect this theoretical direction, and they bring these theories into the world in tangible form, placed underground to grow new directions out of them. On the other hand, the seed paper poems and all the other poems we read and write serve as a bridge between academic discourse and pressing concerns of the public. Poetry, an ancient, primal expression of ideas and images that register in language, if only barely, provides this connective mechanism. In conversation with countless ancient and present-day poets, we seek to add our voices to the re-composition.

REFERENCES

Dungy, Camille. 2009. *Black Nature: Four Centuries of African American Nature Poetry*. Athens: University of Georgia Press.

Food and Agriculture Organization of the United Nations (FAO). n.d. "Key Facts and Findings." Accessed January 5, 2020. http://www.fao.org.

Gay, Ross. 2015. "Catalog of Unabashed Gratitude." Poetry Foundation. https://www.poetryfoundation.org.

Ghosh, Amitav. 2016. *The Great Derangement: Climate Change and the Unthinkable*. Chicago: University of Chicago Press.

Guthman, Julie. 2019. *Wilted: Pathogens, Chemicals, and the Fragile Future of the Strawberry Industry*. Oakland: University of California Press.

Kearney, Douglas. 2015. *Mess and Mess and*. Las Cruces, NM: Noemi.

Kimmerer, Robin Wall. 2013. *Braiding Sweetgrass: Indigenous Wisdom, Scientific Knowledge, and the Teachings of Plants*. Minneapolis, MN: Milkweed.

King, Tiffany Lethabo. 2019. *The Black Shoals: Offshore Formations of Black and Native Studies*. Durham, NC: Duke University Press.

Kirschenmann, Frederick L. 2010. *Cultivating an Ecological Conscience: Essays from a Farmer Philosopher*. Berkeley, CA: Counterpoint.

Lorde, Audre. 1984. *Sister Outsider: Essays and Speeches*. Trumansburg, NY: Crossing.

McLane, Maureen N. 2017. "Plants, Poetics, Possibilities; Or, Two Cheers for Fallacies Especially Pathetic Ones!" *Representations* 140, no. 1 (Fall): 101–20. doi: 10.1525/rep.2017.140.1.101.

McNally, Jess. 2010. "Earth's Most Stunning Fractal Patterns." *Wired*, September 10. https://www.wired.com/.

Nixon, Rob. 2011. *Slow Violence and the Environmentalism of the Poor*. Cambridge, MA: Harvard University Press.

Pollan, Michael. 2013. *Cooked: A Natural History of Transformation*. New York: Penguin.

Posmentier, Sonya. 2017. *Cultivation and Catastrophe: The Lyric Ecology of Modern Black Literature*. Baltimore, MD: Johns Hopkins University Press.

Quashie, Kevin. 2021. *Black Aliveness, or a Poetics of Being*. Durham, NC: Duke University Press.

Rich, Adrienne. 2003. *What Is Found There: Notebooks on Poetry and Politics*. New York: W. W. Norton.

Scigaj, Leonard. 1999. *Sustainable Poetry: Four American Ecopoets*. Lexington: University of Kentucky Press.

United States Department of Agriculture Economic Research Service (USDA). n.d. "Food Security Status of U.S. Households in 2021." Accessed December 13, 2022. https://www.ers.usda.gov.

4

Performance Studies

Brazilian Identity Politics and the Performance of Commensality

SCOTT ALVES BARTON

My multidisciplinary scholarship focusing on African diaspora food-ways as a location of culinary knowledge resides at the confluence of my academic work and my experience as a practicing chef. This essay examines how I came to locate my work at the intersection of academic inquiry and applied public culinary performance, all in the service of illuminating the history and culture of the African diaspora.

I came to this work more as a practitioner than a theorist, having spent three decades as a professional chef, consultant, and culinary educator. I had initially been inspired by my mother, Sylvia Pauline Alves Barton, a Harlemite in the early twentieth century, who had aspired to be a chef, an audacious and absurd option for a woman, even more so for a Black woman, in the late 1930s. Instead, Sylvia became a registered dietitian, a career compromise. Sylvia raised my brother and me in the kitchen, initially using it as an alternative play area in our pre-kindergarten years. As an adolescent I learned recipe development, costing, and technique from my mother, cooking with the same fervor my teen peers poured into their sports competitions. At that time, Blacks, male or female, were infrequently represented in culinary positions of authority. The politics of exclusion caused me to believe that there was no place for someone like me in professional kitchens, forestalling my aspirations as it had done to hers. I was consistently reminded of this by verbal denigration among some of my peers and by invisible ceilings and closed doors for advancement. Later, as a cook, chef, and educator, I experienced the strict hierarchies of knowledge dissemination and teamwork as normative behaviors emanating from the executive chef in a brigade-style kitchen, a practice analogous to Candomblé's *Iyabasses* (post-menopausal woman chef) in sacred kitchens (about which I will have more to say below).

When I made the reflexive turn into research and documentation of enskilled (learned in relation to a more skilled artisan who demonstrates and corrects their embodied knowledge) and intergenerational learning in Brazilian homes and sacred kitchens, I was forced to challenge my own indigenous knowledge. My chef's training had favored Western notions of professionalism, and it was easy to critique certain folk techniques that had been born out of necessity. When and where I could actively listen and eschew the didacticism of my French training, I began to see the excellence and consistency in craft, perseverance, professionalism, and creativity and the intentionality and desire to embrace and honor the bounty of one's larder, reflective of enskilled learning. The sacred and secular kitchens I observed during my fieldwork were organized and maintained by politically and economically marginalized individuals. Decisions about who could touch, butcher, cook, or present each dish followed strict dictums that were based on gender, skill, fealty, levels of advancement, and age in a sacred culinary space.

One of my goals in graduate school had been to apply my culinary skill and knowledge with a theoretical engagement in food studies. Thus, I employed the lenses of anthropology, history, and Africana studies, as well as interdisciplinary study in gender, culture, performance, and religion to better explicate and critique what I saw and experienced in northeastern Brazil. I complemented my work in Brazil with culinary research in Afro-Mexican pueblos and research in Macau, Hong Kong, and Cambodia. These were all locations where food and faith are indelibly linked to cultural identity. Through these experiences, the issues of resistance, power, and hegemony provoked several fundamental research questions. I will first describe my scholarly work in Brazil and then demonstrate the applied nature of my work through three brief vignettes, each illustrating a performative meal, the nourishment of mind, spirit, and body through a repast.

My primary research, titled "Food for the Gods: Sacred Nagô Culinary Religious Culture in Northeastern Brazil," examines the ways in which food is used to negotiate sacred and secular Brazilian African identity. Building on scholarly research in history, anthropology, folklore, and cultural studies, my work identifies food as a marker of cultural and transnational identity with a primary focus on the culinary influences Africans brought to the Americas during the colonial era and their manifestations in contemporary society. I am an ethnographer, supported by other qualitative methods to observe and analyze the roles of gender, race, and food in the sacred prayer rituals and complementary secular culinary activities of women in communities who strongly identify with Nagô (Yoruba) and Candomblé culture in the northeastern Brazilian states of Bahia and Maranhão, as well as in Rio de Janeiro. Candomblé, a diffused monotheistic religion honoring a diverse community of divinities, is dominated by ideologies of the Yoruba, the last and largest group of enslaved West Africans imported to Brazil.

Through a detailed study of the *banquete sagrado da comida de santo*, a multicourse banquet prepared by women for the sixteen primary deities of the Nagô pantheon, as well as other important food-centered rituals and practices, my work documents historic culinary markers of the African presence and analyzes their level of cultural importance in secular foods and sacred offerings. My findings create an assessment of patterns of use and current relevance to women in Afro-Brazilian communities in the northeastern region. Part of the research involves a film component, which complements the written text of these important food rituals and practices and adds a living, breathing dimension to the descriptive and analytical work.

Food is everywhere in worship but underdeveloped as a focus in religious scholarship. In most Western societies, the overt associations of food and spirituality have diminished, other than as direct victuals of communion. Coke and Pepsi drinkers, for example, are unaware of the sacred implications inscribed in the culture and consumption of kola nuts established in West Africa. Similarly, on New Year's Day, American southerners prepare Hoppin' John, a pilaf of black-eyed peas and rice, without any awareness of the dish's currency as a potential offering for West African deities. My research considers twenty-three such dishes located on a continuum of sacred to secular, which contribute to both individual and community identity politics and by extension to the perception of Afro-Brazilians by other Brazilians, foreigners, and tourists, from the colonial era to the present day. This dialectic directly affects the consciousness and lived experience of my respondents, whether or not they practice Candomblé (Olga and Lima 2010; Rodrigues 1932).

The study vividly illustrates the relevance of food as a foundational aspect of religious practice and cultural identity and contributes to scholarship regarding food, religion, ethnicity, and identity for Brazilians of African ancestry, as well as to African diaspora studies in general. In so doing, it demonstrates food studies as a fruitful mode of inquiry for academic scholarship (Black Public Sphere Collective 1995, 4–39; Hall 1996). The dishes making up the *banquete sagrado da comida de santo*, including the labor that cultivates the ingredients and prepares the finished dishes, identifies indigenous knowledge, enskilled labor, and the advancement of culinary cultural and spiritual traditions that originated in West Africa, as well as the influence of Native and European cultural heritage. The long historical connections, however, have been slow to emerge in academic scholarship (Carney 2011; Crosby 2003).

Upon my arrival in Brazil, I immediately became aware of my local respondents' view of me as yet another African American embracing Afro-Brazilian culture to find their "roots." This perception forced me to be both introspective and reflexive in my approach to the work and to those who became my interlocutors. My core area of interest became cloistered religious communities and home kitchens steeped in secret knowledge. This secret knowledge, I learned, was parsed out slowly over decades based on qualities that included trustworthiness, status within one's religious community, and an aspirational commitment to religious dogma, as well as class, personal pride, and privacy. Not having been raised in either a Catholic or the Yoruba/Bantu (Yorubana) matrix of religious traditions, I had to quickly adapt. I labored to learn the community's core values, understand the identity and agency of Catholic saints and West African *orixá* (gods), and the quotidian practices associated with each religion and to grasp the unique West African vocabularies embedded in Brazilian-Portuguese linguistics related to foodstuffs, gastronomy, and religious values.

To best comprehend my respondents, I realized I needed to understand their historical marginality, the result of a history of foreign researchers' interpretations, assumptions, and essentialization of their culture and its religion. I needed to comprehend the community's reactions to these intrusions, which included fostering self-reinvention to better represent themselves, counter misrepresentations, and improve their status and perception in and outside of their communities.

Epistemologically, I understood that researching marginalized individuals and alternative religions required particular attention to my subjects (Clifford 2022; Ortner 1995). This is further complicated by the fact that African diaspora history is based in orality, not the written word. Therefore, when we can uncover any thoughts, ideas, or writings that underscore the importance of marginalized people who have explicitly been written out of the archives, we need to add their voices to the archive, critically read existing archives against the grain, or establish new, more inclusive archives. For instance, the *baianas de acarajé*, (Bahian black-eyed pea fritter vendors) and their antecedents, *as ganhadeiras*, the enslaved and free women of color as itinerant day laborers, laundresses, and street-food vendors, are ubiquitous markers of West African heritage. These subsistence cottage-industry entrepreneurs akin to market women on the continent are emblems of corporeal archives existent in the bodies and lifeworlds of these street vendors in the Brazilian public sphere. As such, their somatic knowledge is fundamental as a research focus.

The Bahian streets, whether colonial and populated by slaves, free people of color, and white Portuguese businessmen or in the current multiracial economically and politically divisive society, can be seen as a site of multiple public spheres. The *baiana's barraca* kiosk is viewed as the repository of an alternative archive of African diaspora culture, and culinary knowledge is constituted by common exchanges of everyday people frequently written out of historical narratives. Or, to quote Nigerian author Chinua Achebe, "Until the lions have their own historians, the history of the hunt will always glorify the hunter." These subordinate social groups (sacred and profane) who constitute alternative public spheres create and circulate new narrative discourses in the process of producing and consuming the foods peddled by the *baianas*. This allows the victual linguistic discourse to develop opposing constructions of identity and cultural orientation that chart a trajectory of diasporic consciousness where food is the mediator of identity politics.

At all junctures of my work, the problematic issue of authenticity arose, as if one could easily spot the "authentic" as a universal concept or material manifestation of alleged cultural purity and linear origin. The supposed authentic could be interpreted distinctly by different interlocutors in and outside of my research communities. Given the alleged ambiguity of orality and the voice of marginalized people in a world that privileges written texts and elite discourses, who decides what or whose cultural knowledge and foodways are "authentic"? In a relatively homogenous community, which recipe is authentic, or most authentic, became an ongoing question. Consider the basic recipe for the unctuous condiment *vatapá*, a puree of cashews, peanuts, smoked and dried shrimp, and palm oil bound with various thickeners, most typically bread/breadcrumbs or *farinha de mandioca* (manioc flour), ground jackfruit seeds, pureed breadfruit, rice flour, or yams (Barton 2010–12; Vianna 1940, 70). Most of the binders refer directly to European colonial influence. Which, then, best reflects West African cookery?

Melville Herskovits theorized about the acculturation of "authentic" behaviors and cultural transference from the continent to the Americas predicated on his ideas of syncretic behavior within a religio-cultural dialectic. He troubled prior reductive and/or racist readings of West African cultural, religious, and culinary norms built solely overtop of Catholic traditions, without appreciating how culinary traditions along with religious and other epistemes are frequently derived from an amalgam of inspirations and cultural confluences born on the continent pre-contact (Herskovits 1941, xxii–ii; Stewart and Shaw 2005).

I further sharpened my cognitive understanding of the authentic by placing Herskovits in conversation with James Clifford's ideas of cultural interpretation/translation and Sherry Ortner's concept of "practice theory," those somatic embedded-knowledge practices consociated within a fictive or non-fictive kin group as a network of social structures, lifestyles, and group dynamics that embody dissent, everyday forms of resistance, and the power of refusal. For example, in classic carnival performances, costumes obscure gender and race, and costumed individuals frequently throw their voices to obscure their identity. Their fictionalized identities enable them to confront people in higher-class positions, individuals who have victimized them, or those whom they desire and to speak freely and bluntly without fear of retribution. This is demonstrated in Bakhtin's carnivalesque theories where the "lower bodily stratum" can assert itself, literally and figuratively, and react to or contest hegemonic power (Clifford 2002, 21–54; Ortner 2008, 1–9, 155).

In Afro-Brazilian Candomblé religious communities where sacred dishes are prepared to be virtually consumed by ostensibly attendant deities, I learned that the *iyalorixá* or *babalorixá* (high priestess/priest) employed cowrie shell divination to see if the *orixá* (deities) were pleased with a given offering. I was always assured that the offerings, *ebó*, were accepted. And when substitutions were made based on availability of foodstuffs or community economics, the dedicated adhesion to protocol of the cooks was understood and appreciated by the gods. Authenticity became relative, particularly if we interrogate ingredients available on the continent and those adopted via the Columbian Exchange and the realities of availability due to climate and the Middle Passage. Corn, native to the Americas and adopted into the African diaspora pantry, becomes inculcated as a sacred food. Bright red *dendê* palm oil, a sacred African ingredient, was not native to the Americas, necessitating the use of annatto oil to redden such foods as Gullah red rice (Barton 2010–15).

The multicourse *banquete sagrado da comida de santo* is but one example of a repast as a *lieux de memoire*, a meal that is a site of memory and profound center of commensality that has a global cultural resonance. The poetics of the meal event is a culturally significant moment in the "food-ritual-memory" dialectic as symbolic ritual practice is transcribed on top of everyday existence. Dishes such as *acarajé*, black-eyed pea fritters, for example, while mundane street food in one context, take on intense religious and ritualistic meaning in another. Acarajé purchased at a corner *barraca*, split in half and filled with *molho pimenta* (hot sauce), *vatapá*, sautéed shrimp, and a chopped salad of tomatoes and onions is an adequate lunch or a hearty snack. In a sacred context, it becomes something entirely different. In this setting. it is served uncut until presented in offering by a priestess/priest or served in conjunction with a number of other dishes. Here, *acarajé* becomes linked to ancestral traditions and an acknowledgement of faith in West African/Candomblé dogma.

The commensal meal is a ritual activity that is enacted across cultures, geographies, and time yet holds similarities in meanings and purpose for the diverse communities of respondents, diners, and collaborators. The performative meals I participated in, described below in short vignettes, are in direct conversation with my research in Brazil. The research, development, and staging of the events function as critical commemorations and as interventions for participants, audiences, and communities at large. Such performative meals also illuminate multisensory aspects. The ability to embrace gaps in the historical narrative with embodied practice, for example, may help complete or complement some of the narratives and to better situate identity politics, knowledge formation, and culinary traditions, particularly within an African diaspora context (Carney and Rosomoff 2011; Hartman 2008; hooks 2015; Ortner 1995; Sharpe 2016).

These recent meals examine questions of community, identity, politics, marginalization, enskilled women's work, and applied practice as a reflection of food and foodways. My goal in each performative repast was to interrogate the engagement across difference to develop a more comprehensive and less idealized interpretation of a social group other than my own or to formulate a better contextual understanding of my own diaspora. I begin with my annual work as a public scholar at Lynden Sculpture Garden.

VIGNETTE #1: IMAGINING LIZZIE THROUGH *ELIZA'S CABINET OF CURIOSITIES TO JUBA—SANCTUARY (2016–19)*

Music, spoken word, culinary, and spiritual performances in the Lynden Sculpture Gardens of Milwaukee, commemorating cultural connections to land, women's knowledge, histories of enslavement, and rice agriculture.

Where your ancestors do not live, you cannot build your house.
—Kongo proverb

Building on the history and the agricultural legacy of enslaved African provision gardens that dotted plantation slave quarters, this multidisciplinary performative project in Milwaukee imagined an emancipation garden of a semifictional character, Eliza (Lizzie). Lizzie is an amalgam of artist and professor Portia Cobb's Gullah-Geechee ancestors who worked the land for generations. Sculptor, educator, and designer Folayemi "Fo" Wilson created the installation *Eliza's Cabinet of Curiosities*, a full-scale structure that is both *Wunderkammer* and slave cabin. Wilson designed the installation to represent what a nineteenth-century woman of African descent might have collected in her living quarters. In the summer of 2016, Cobb and I occupied the structure to illuminate Lizzie, Eliza's field-slave counterpart. The work was concurrently an actual garden and a historical-performative project that engaged oral history, video, and performance (Lyndon Sculpture Garden 2016).

Juba dis and Juba dat, and Juba killed da yellow cat
You sift the meal and ya gimme the husk, you bake the bread and ya
    gimme the crust
You eat the meat and ya gimme the skin, and that's the way, my
    mama's troubles begin.
Kongo song/dance

My work was an homage and re-memorialization of the "20 and odd Africans" who landed at the Jamestown River Colony, Virginia Commonwealth, August 20, 1619. Culinarily, *Eliza's Cabinet of Curiosities, Juba—Sanctuary* (Juba 2016) featured rice, a sacred and secular foodstuff for the Mende (one of the two largest ethnolinguistic groups in Sierra Leone and expert rice cultivators) and Low Country peoples, and a throughline of diaspora foodways and knowledge in the Gullah-Geechee Heritage Corridor of the Low Country. Rice agriculture and women's work symbolized the imagined home and life of fictional enslaved woman Lizzie. *Eliza's Cabinet of Curiosities, Juba—Sanctuary* acknowledged a collective past as a reimagined visceral reality. Particular focus was given to the labor and knowledge of African descendant women, giving voice to our ancestral past and current lifeworlds.

Employing my skills both as a chef and scholar of African diaspora foodways, for the performance I baked and served *philpy*, a nineteenth-century Low Country rice bread, and hybrid *acaça agidi*, traditionally a hominy mush steamed in a banana leaf that is a primary offertory food for West African deities (*agidi* is rice based; here, the *acaça agidi* was made of rice and corn). We also served watermelon sorrel, or *bissap*. By either name (one Caribbean, the other West African), this spiced and sweetened hibiscus tea is often spiked with rum and historically reserved for celebrations. My Bajan American mother, Sylvia, made it frequently during the holidays of my youth.

The Bantu/Yoruba use of the word *juba* directly emanates from rice culture, the term coming from the plant tassels, "a sparsed juba, or tuft" (1688). From Sierra Leone to Charleston to Milwaukee, we celebrate rice culture, Africana indigenous knowledge, and skill at the hearth. Further, *juba*, or "to *juber*," is an ecstatic syncopated West African jig marked by hand, knee, and thigh slapping with stomping of feet on the floor. In the diaspora, from *juba* comes the term *jubilee*, a release, a season of rejoicing and celebration (Lawal 2005, 291–98). To be in conversation with Fo Wilson's *Eliza's Peculiar Cabinet of Curiosities, Juba—Sanctuary* affords a moment to *juba*, to jubilee. A safe haven. August 20, 2019, was the four hundredth anniversary of the arrival of "20 odd Negros" landing in the Jamestown, Virginia, colony as enslaved. To commemorate this moment, I performed as an Afro-futurist griot in conversation and performance with Vi Hawkins, the founding member of the Jazzy Jewels, and her group of septuagenarian and octogenarian Great Migrator women "cheerleaders," community leaders, and advocates for women's rights (WTMJ Radio 2010). Each of the six Jazzy Jewels represented archetypical skills and knowledge centers that African-descendant women had had. The performance, sung and spoken, rendered quotidian women's work visible in plain sight (Lyndon Sculpture Garden 2019).

For the performance space, I was able to obtain Moruga Hill upland red bearded rice seed from Trinidadian anthropologist Francis Morean to grow in Lizzie's garden (Severson 2018). This seed was purported to be a West African strain passed intergenerationally since colonialism. Having taken a year to acquire, it was planted at an inopportune moment in the Wisconsin growing cycle. Still, it took, flowered, and gave forth more seed before being wintered over in a greenhouse. While subsequent DNA analysis has questioned its African provenance, the acquisition and performance did provoke a fertile discourse within the community of artists, growers, immigrants, and the general public familiar with Lynden and the cabin.

In addition to collaborating with Portia Cobb, over my two-year summer residency I worked with a dozen Great Migrator men and women originally from Alabama, Arkansas, Louisiana, and Mississippi who ranged in age between sixty and their late nineties. Some had begun working the fields or in kitchens as young as nine years of age. Through the interactions, many of the same themes emerged that informed my work in Brazil, Mexico, and Asia, including the importance of female age rank and status, culinary enskillment, and the passing on of culinary traditions within working class/working poor households. Serendipitously, my preparation of nineteenth-century Low Country menus for these elders triggered a heady exchange of knowledge and memories. They were accustomed to similar ingredients but very different resulting recipes and meals. In addition, the gustatory and technical distinctions developed trust based on their appreciation of my culinary acumen. Overall, the experiences generated a profound sense of community.

VIGNETTE #2: RE: PAST: MALAGA ISLAND, MAINE (JULY 12, 2018)

A performative dinner commemorating July 1, 1912, when forty-seven mixed-race members of the community were evicted, some institutionalized, to make way for a resort that never materialized.

On Malaga Island, on lace clothed tables set with antique mismatched china and wildflower bouquets, we were fed a supper typical of an early twentieth-century subsistence fishing community: dry hopped cider, sun tea, salmon and salt-cod chowder, chow-chow, Marfax beans with salt pork belly, summer berry pudding, and Abenaki corn molasses bread. All foods were locally grown and sourced, served on antique plates, and laden with symbolic meanings of people, ethnicity and place. Lobstermen in their working boats had ferried groups of six to eight individuals from Phippsburg to Malaga Island, in Casco Bay, Maine, on July 12, a sunny Thursday afternoon. Professor Myron Beasley invited us to "commemorate and remember the people of Malaga at a performative dinner—a re: past." Each of us was the cipher for one of the forty-seven members of the humble fishing community of Black, white and mixed-race peoples.

In 1911, after purchasing the island for $473, the state of Maine sold it to cronies of Governor Frederick W. Plaisted. On July 1, 1912, the residents were forcibly evicted. Families were separated, and some residents were institutionalized at the newly opened Maine School for the Feeble-Minded. Plaisted's friend, Dr. Gustavus Kilgore, had signed the commitment orders for the islanders to allow a developer to build a resort, although the resort never materialized. The island had (and has) four working wells providing fresh water, making it an ideal site for development. The houses on the forty-one-acre island at the mouth of the New Meadows River were leveled, the schoolhouse removed, graves exhumed, and remains not lost were piled into mass unmarked graves. The island has since remained deserted, bringing new, uncanny meaning to Maine's nickname of "Vacationland."

Re: Past's dining guests included the island's descendants, food scholars, historians, archaeologists, rangers, farmers, and elected officials.

Assisting the performative rite of eviction were our waiters, Phippsburg High School theatre and art students supervised by Bates College theater department faculty. Before the archetypical houses built in situ were disassembled and carted off, the students re-created conversations from the historical record. Each of us called out the name of one of the residents, and we consumed our "Re: Past." Hymns and spirituals were sung poetry read; memorialization of the lives and livelihoods lost and testimonies of living descendants highlighted the event. It was a celebration of unforgetting (Barton 2019).

VIGNETTE #3: KINSTON, NC, END OF SEASON DINNER
FOR THE PBS SERIES A CHEF'S LIFE (OCTOBER 22, 2018)

A Chef's Life "Final Harvest" episode celebratory dinner

To end its six-season run, the Peabody Award–winning documentary-style cooking series, *A Chef's Life*, hosted a "Cast Supper." We were approximately thirty at one long, wooden table built for the occasion. Three generations of Black and white southerners and northerners ate Sam Jones's whole-hog barbeque, which was finished in front of us, accompanied by freshly baked cornbread, chow-chow, and oversized platters of grilled vegetables culled from Warner Brothers Farm, along with deep-fried turkey rillettes, baked field peas, personal paw-paw puddings with vanilla wafers and sesame crumble, and wine and beer. Bringing together featured chef Vivian Howard's "family of choice" at one grand harvest table, folks who had shaped the television show's success, as well as that of Vivian's eponymous restaurant, The Chef and the Farmer, seemed fitting and appropriate.

The cast included farmers, provisioners, cooks, food writers, kinfolk, and chefs like me who had been guests, teachers, mentors, or willing customers at chef Vivian Howard's and documentary filmmaker Cynthia Hill's television table. This "Final Harvest" episode took place on Howard-family land at dusk, in a cloistered acre shrouded in silage, corn drying on the stalk, to later serve as winter animal feed. We were served a local late September eastern North Carolina bounty produced by farmers and chefs who had contributed their skills and knowledge over the last several years. For a brief moment, we lived off and savored the "fat of the land" (Hill et al. 2017).

Conclusion

These staged culinary events highlight a developing, performative turn in some of my research. Each commensal meal featured public-facing components that combined academic and public audiences and fostered an experiential engagement with food. Experiential engagement with food and foodways seems a natural progression for me following decades of work as an executive chef. Restaurant work and even more so catering are theatrical performances. For both the cook and the waiter, restaurant work is a daily staged performance, from the rising tension during the prep period to the notes given during staff meal, the "opening of the house," service itself, and the final notes, often over a staff beverage. As with professional theatre, in restaurants price identifies audience and access. The events discussed above involved invited guests as both actors and bystanders or were fully open to the public. I believe that by harnessing theory to applied practice as a literal and symbolic reference to historical narratives provides an opportunity to expand the appreciation of food studies as a relevant discipline and method of research and to increase interaction between academic and general audiences. Specifically, as evidenced with the recent premier of Terence Blanchard's *Fire up in My Bones*, the Metropolitan Opera's first opera by a Black composer, Black culture expressed performatively as a politics of identity and *site of memory* provides a corrective to prior discriminatory historical narratives of my culture.

One of my key research questions has been how the performance of commensality, while harnessed with a political or sociocultural intent, can have resonance for the diners and community at large beyond self-aggrandizement. All the above-mentioned endeavors—my work at Lynden, the Malaga *Re: Past* project, or *A Chef's Life*—and my foundational work in Brazil are meals that explore these contradictions and tensions. Symbolically, this commensal moment is often held in celebration to honor individuals, communities, or important events, transforming the simple act of ingestion to one where favored food of the honored are prepared for them, or as a memory of their legacy. By consuming foods that refer to individuals within the social group, the guests metaphorically consume the spirit of that person, embodied by foods that they favored or excelled in preparing, thereby recalling their contribution to the community as a shared public act. Similarly, when consecrated as an act of memorialization for the deceased, repasts as an acknowledgment of the dead in a public sphere also allow the living to exist without the need to exert effort as they grieve and appreciate the life that now exists as memory. My work at its core considers everyday meals, religious offerings, and funerary repasts in an Afro-diaspora context, where honoring our elders and the departed ancestors who exist among us requires (and allows us the privilege) engagement with traditional African religious dogma (Barton 2019).

REFERENCES

Alaketu, Olga de, and Vivaldo da Costa Lima. 2010. *A Comida de Santo Numa Casa de Queto da Bahía*. São Paulo: Corrupio.

Bakhtin, Mikhail M. 1968. *Rabelais and His World*. Cambridge, MA: MIT Press.

Bakhtin, Mikhail, and Michael Holquist. 1981. *The Dialogic Imagination: Four Essays*. Austin: University of Texas Press.

Barton, Scott Alves. 2010–12. Ethnographic interviews with various iyalorixá, babalorixá, and storytellers in Bahia and Maranhão. Copy in author's possession.

———. 2016. "Juba: Sanctuary." *Academia*. https://www.academia.edu

———. 2019. "Repasting: A Metonymy." *Liminalities* 15 (2): 1–19. http://liminalities.net/15-2/metonymy.pdf.

Black Public Sphere Collective. 1995. *The Black Public Sphere: A Public Culture Cook*. Chicago: University of Chicago Press.

Carney, Judith Ann, and Richard Nicholas Rosomoff. 2011. *In the Shadow of Slavery: Africa's Botanical Legacy in the Atlantic World*. Berkeley: University of California Press.

Clifford, James. 2002. *The Predicament of Culture: Twentieth-Century Ethnography, Literature, and Art*. Cambridge, MA: Harvard University Press.

Crosby, Alfred W. 2003. *The Columbian Exchange: Biological and Cultural Consequences of 1492*. Westport, CT: Praeger.

Grosvenor, Vertamae Smart. 1970. "Kitchen Crisis." In *The Black Woman: An Anthology*, edited by Toni Cade Bambara, 119–23. New York: Washington Square.

Hall, Stuart, and Paul Du Gay. 1996. *Questions of Cultural Identity*. Thousand Oaks, CA: Sage.

Hartman, Saidiya. 2008. "Venus in Two Acts." *Small Axe* 26:1–14.

Herskovits, Melville J. (1941) 1990 . *The Myth of the Negro Past*. New York: Harper & Brothers. Reprint, Boston: Beacon Press.

Hill, Cynthia, Vivian Howard, Amy Schumaker, and Ben Knight. 2017. *A Chef's Life*. Season 5, special final episode. PBS TV. https://www.pbs.org.

Holm, Randle. 1688. *The Academy of Armory; Or, A Storehouse of Armory and Blazon*. 1st ed. Chester: Self-published.

hooks, bell. 2015. "Eating the Other: Desire and Resistance." In *Black Looks: Race and Representation*, 21–40. Boston: South End.

Juba Sanctuary. 2016. https://www.academia.edu/55517598/JUBA_SANCTUARY.

Koster, Henry. 1816. *Travels in Brazil*. London: Printed for Longman, Hurst, Rees, Orme, and Brown.

Lawal, Babatunde. 2005. "Reclaiming the Past: Yoruba Elements in African American Arts." In *The Yoruba Diaspora in the Atlantic World*, edited by Toyin Falola and Matt D. Childs, 291–324. Bloomington: Indiana University Press.

Lyndon Sculpture Garden. 2016. "Imagining Eliza and Lizzie: The Garden Project with Scott Barton and Portia Cobb." Lyndon Sculpture Garden. https://www.lyndenscul pturegarden.org.

———. 2019. "Performance on the Porch: Scott Barton: Juba—Sanctuary." Lyndon Sculpture Garden. https://www.lyndensculpturegarden.org.

Lynn, Martin.1997. *Commerce and Economic Change in West Africa: The Palm Oil Trade in the Nineteenth Century*. Cambridge, UK: Cambridge University Press.

Ortner, Sherry B. 1995. "Resistance and the problem of ethnographic refusal." *Comparative Studies in Society and History*, no. 37: 173–93.

———. 2008. *Anthropology and Social Theory: Culture, Power, and the Acting Subject*. Durham, NC: Duke University Press.

Pálsson, Gísli. 1994. "Enskilment at Sea Man." *Journal of the Royal Anthropological Institute*. 29 (4). https://notendur.hi.is.

Ripert, Eric, and Veronica Chambers. 2017. *32 Yolks: From My Mother's Table to Working the Line*. New York: Random House.

Rodrigues, Nina Raymundo. 1932. *Os Africanos no Brasil*. São Paulo: Companhia Editora Nacional.

Severson, Kim. 2018. "Finding a Lost Strain of Rice, and Clues to Slave Cooking." *New York Times*, February 13. https://www.nytimes.com.

Sharpe, Christina. 2016. *In the Wake: On Blackness and Being*. Durham, NC: Duke University Press.

Stewart, Charles, and Rosalind Shaw. 2005. *Syncretism / Anti-syncretism: The Politics of Religious Synthesis*. London: Routledge.

Sutton, David Evan. 2006. *Remembrance of Repasts: An Anthropology of Food and Memory*. Oxford: Berg.

Vianna, Sodré. 1940. *Caderno de Xangô: 50 Receitas da Cosinha Bahiana do Litoral e do Nordeste: Uma Reportagem de Sodré Vianna*. Bahia: Livraria Editora Bahiana.

Wetherell, James, and William Hadfield. 1860. *Brazil: Stray Notes from Bahia: Being Extracts from Letters During a Residence of Fifteen years*. Liverpool: Webb and Hunt.

Wilson, Folayemi (Fo). 2016. "Eliza's Peculiar Cabinet of Curiosities." Lynden Sculpture Garden, Milwaukee, WI. https://www.fowilson.com/projects/elizas-peculiar-cabi net-of-curiosities.

WTMJ Radio. 2010. "Positively Milwaukee: WTMJ4 Interviews the Jazzy Jewels." https://www.youtube.com/watch?v=7A3tConJeag.

Health, Nutrition, and the Culinary Arts

The second section, "Health, Nutrition, and the Culinary Arts," turns its attention to engagement with individual and communal health through the lenses of public health and nutrition, highlighting the relevance of food for both personal well-being and social dimensions such as justice, equity, and sustainability. It also focuses on the culinary arts and the role that recipes play in bringing food to the table, reminding us that the materiality of what we grow, process, prepare, and eat is central to food studies.

Moving beyond its traditional grounding in the humanities and soft social sciences and into the realms of nutrition and public health proved to be a maturing moment for NYU food studies. As mentioned earlier, the first decade of food studies (1996–2006) established itself as a legitimate field within academia, while its second decade (2006–) demonstrated that scholars who identified with it were able to produce interesting and important research in a multidisciplinary dialogue with health scholars and professionals. This was an important, and perhaps inevitable, step given our close proximity to the NYU nutrition and public health programs. This unique department composition (food studies + nutrition + public health) for better or worse aligned three methodologically and epistemologically diverse programs of study together, and while it was difficult at times to create robust academic conversations, the interactions and attempts to find common ground led to fruitful interchange.

Health and medicine as fields of knowledge and practice have been around for a long time, taking different forms as human understanding about the body evolved and changed and also differing across cultures. The study of nutrition—eating and drinking for optimal health—was first (logically) embedded in the flora and fauna of the natural world. In the eighteenth and nineteenth centuries, as advances in chemistry revealed microscopic building blocks, the study and practice of nutrition transformed into what was later termed *nutritionism*, the assumption that the chemical values in food equal or surpass food's holistic value. Thus, the academic study of nutrition falls within a science-based approach to generating and evaluating data, with its emphasis on the scientific method: observation, experimentation, measurement, replication, and hypothesis formation. Public health as an academic field is relatively new, formalized in the nineteenth century as scientific experiments improving municipal water and sanitation proved crucial to human well-being, among other endeavors. Itself an interdisciplinary field, public health comprises disciplines in the sciences (epidemiology, biostatistics) and the social sciences (sociology, policy, psychology).

The academic streaming of the culinary arts features another trajectory altogether. Cooking programs, emerging mostly in trade-oriented community colleges and culinary schools, were regarded as alternatives to college training. Universities had developed hospitality programs, featuring hotel management and the restaurant industry but more focused on the financial and operations sides. Cooking courses tended to belong in home economic programs. Prior to NYU food studies, as described in earlier chapters, the NYU department housed programs in home economics, nutrition, and hotel and restaurant management. In the late twentieth century, thanks to the rise of fine dining as entertainment and of food-related media on television, professional cooking became elevated in status, and chefs became celebrities. Food and food work gained importance and cultural cache.

One of the goals of NYU food studies, as Marion Nestle and her early collaborators envisioned it, was to bring serious attention to food into the program—to go beyond home economics' emphasis on micro- and macronutrients and embrace food aesthetics, tastes, and techniques. Instead of focusing on the elevated aspects of food, food studies sought to tie culinary techniques and ingredients to cultural identity, historical evolution, and issues of social justice and sustainability.

In this section, authors demonstrate how the primarily humanities/social sciences approach of NYU food studies (employing cultural, social, and historical perspectives) can provide insight when applied to fields and disciplines in other domains: nutrition (within the sciences), public health (straddling the sciences and social sciences), and the culinary arts (part of the hospitality industry).

5

Public Health

A Food Studies Perspective on Policymaking and Policy Analysis

BETH C. WEITZMAN

In this chapter, I consider how adopting a food studies lens, with its greater attention to culture, aesthetics, history, and the food system as a whole, might facilitate the creation of more impactful food policies, especially in regard to health outcomes. A food studies lens also encourages thinking beyond what is purchased, cooked, and consumed to incorporate what is grown and what is wasted. Food policy could be strengthened by opening the lens to see a greater diversity of perspectives and issues.

I begin this chapter with a brief description of my scholarly background and how I came to refocus my attention from other health policy issues to food policy. This is followed by a discussion of how and why food policy has become so central to the field of health policy. I then turn my attention to specific food policies aimed at improving the public's health and examine how a food studies lens might offer a critique and a strengthening of these policies and approaches.

How I Came to Food Policy

How can public policies be used to improve the health and well-being of the American people, especially for those communities with the greatest needs? This question motivated my graduate training and my first decades as a professor and researcher in the field of public policy. Trying to answer that question required the development of a tool kit of both quantitative and qualitative research skills and the flexible use of theories borrowed from several social science disciplines. The breadth of the question took me down a variety of streets and alleys. It led me to look at the relationship between health and housing and how public policies might be used to reduce homelessness and ameliorate its effects on both physical and mental health. It led me to consider child and youth-centered policies and how they might influence both health and educational outcomes. Government decisions about after-school programs, services to pregnant teens, and youth safety all received my attention as I evaluated policies and programs that might improve the public's health, even as they might fall outside of traditional health-care services. But it would be almost twenty years before I turned my attention to the role of food in health and began to consider the degree to which dietary choices are influenced by the food environment and how this environment may be shaped and reshaped through public policy.

As a scholar focused on the impact of public policies on the health of Americans, my journey into the food arena is far from unique. It is part of an unmistakable trend evidenced by the number of research articles focused on diet, the food environment, and health recently published in respected health policy journals. A recent JSTOR search of journals and books in health policy, public health, and public administration indicated that the number of publications that included discussion of food, health, and policy more than doubled in the decades 1990–2000 and 2010–20. This trend has been amplified by the COVID-19 pandemic, which shined a sharp light on the importance of the food system to societal well-being. Further, large and prestigious health foundations are funding relevant studies, pushing for important changes in food policies and trying to identify strategies to create healthier food environments at the community level. For example, the Robert Wood Johnson Foundation, the nation's largest foundation focused exclusively on health, has in recent years funded a broad program of research concerning healthy food access in their efforts to address the underlying social determinants of health and reduce childhood obesity (RWJF). The New York State Health Foundation has recently made "healthy foods, healthy lives" one if its priority areas (NYSHF). Similarly, state and local governments are experimenting with a wide variety of programs to encourage healthier eating patterns at schools and communities.

All that said, there continues to be a great divide between those of us who entered the food space from the land of health policy and those scholars who have long seen food as a focus for exploring cultural identity, artistic expression, and historic trends. Using the *New York Times* as a metaphor, their section "Science Times" appears on Tuesday and includes numerous articles on the relationship of food, food policy, and health. Wednesday's paper features the "Food" section, replete with food photos, dining and cooking trends past and present, and reviews of restaurants and food purveyors, as well as an increased focus on the struggles faced by the industry and its workers as a result of COVID. Yet there has been little recognition in the articles of the relationship between these two sections and their respective themes, just as there continues to be only the most limited crosspollination in these two scholarly worlds. Might food policy be strengthened by reading both the "Health Science" and "Food" sections?

How Food Policy Became Health Policy

For most of human history, population health was challenged by malnutrition and dietary deficiencies. Over the course of the past one hundred or so years, industrialization, changing demographics, and scientific advances turned this relationship between food and health on its head. Diseases of insufficiency have been replaced by conditions of plenty throughout most of the world. Beginning in the most affluent nations but rapidly spreading to all but the poorest, an overabundance of relatively inexpensive and often highly processed food has greatly contributed to dramatic increases in rates of obesity and the spread of chronic diseases, including many cancers and cardiovascular disease. Large-sample and long-term epidemiological research has made abundantly clear that diet is significantly contributing to poor health outcomes. The Framingham Heart Study, begun in 1948 and continuing to this day, has repeatedly underscored the connection between dietary and other behaviors to health (Hajar 2016).

The costs associated with these diseases, for actual health care but also in lost earnings and reduced abilities, are more frequently borne by the public coffers, making evident that population health is a public good. Beginning in Germany in the late nineteenth century, social insurance programs began shifting the costs of illness and old age, including both lost wages and health care, away from the individual household to the larger community (Social Security Administration n.d.). In the

United States, beginning with the New Deal of the 1930s and greatly expanding in the mid-1960s with the Great Society, federal and state governments became increasingly responsible for the costs associated with disease and disability. These costs represent a significant share of the economy. Prior to COVID-19, nearly 18 percent of the US gross domestic product went to health care, and 45 percent of those costs were paid by federal, state, and local governments (Centers for Medicare and Medicaid Services n.d.). With this financial reality, governments' motivation to identify more effective and efficient approaches to reducing health-care costs crystalized.

This changing context has resulted in a slow but ultimately dramatic shift in how we understand disease prevention. When we think about health policy, whether domestically or globally, we are far more likely to think about health insurance, health organizations, and health-care training than about diets and food choices and the myriad policies that influence them. In recent decades, however, increasing attention has been given to the underlying social determinants of health, which have been estimated to be of far greater importance than health care itself in shaping morbidity and mortality. Behaviors like smoking, excessive drinking, and lack of physical activity have been found to play a larger role in premature death than genetics or health care, and yet individually oriented downstream approaches to changing those behaviors have yielded frustratingly small changes. As a result, researchers and policymakers have increasingly turned their lens upstream to the social determinants of health, such as housing, education, and public safety; there has been a growing recognition within health policy debates of the importance of community and culture in shaping individual behavior. The Robert Wood Johnson Foundation, for example, speaks now of moving communities and organizations toward a "national Culture of Health" (RWJF).

This new focus on the social determinants of health, combined with the increasing salience of dietary-related diseases, has highlighted the importance of the food environment, that is, the political, economic, geographic, and cultural context that shape individuals' dietary options. If we are to use public policy to reshape our diets to promote health, we must turn our attention to the world beyond laboratory science and clinical nutrition to the places in which food choices are made.

History is filled with examples of public policies that have been aimed at ensuring America's access to safe and sufficient food. Indeed, some of the greatest successes in government health interventions fall under this safe-and-sufficient-food umbrella, demonstrating how public policy can help improve the population's health. Public health policies, for example, have contributed to dramatic reductions in morbidity and mortality through improved safety in food processing, dietary supplementation, and clear food labels and honest food advertising (CDC 1998). Other examples include required vitamin D supplementation of milk, safe handling of meats and dairy products throughout the food systems, and local laws governing sanitation in restaurants and retail outlets.

The creation and successful implementation of these policies have not, however, been the product of science alone. Rather, new knowledge regarding nutrition and infectious diseases was turned into policy through the collective action of a host of political players and activists. Upton Sinclair's, *The Jungle* brought public attention to the conditions of the slaughterhouse; only then could the needs of workers and consumers be better balanced against the interests of the meatpacking industry (USFDA 2018). Throughout, public health researchers have advanced the relevant science but it required coalitions and partners in political advocacy to make change possible when food industry interests stood in powerful opposition. Marion Nestle's *Food Politics* (2002) brought new attention to the intensively political nature of food policies. Her analyses have repeatedly underscored the strength of industry lobbyists and interests in limiting government intervention within the food environment.

Of note, members of the public health community have long been interested in the environmental impacts of farming, including pesticide exposures for farm workers; these environmental concerns have infrequently been tied, however, to those associated with diet or even a safe food supply. Rarely has public policy been used to reshape the supply of food—that is, what is grown—to enable healthier eating. Within the worlds of public health and health policy, questions of what we eat have not been well tied to those of what is grown (Neff et al. 2015). Indeed, current dietary guidelines for healthy eating cannot be achieved given current production of fruits and vegetables (Buzby 2006).

Beyond the above-noted efforts to improve food sanitation, dietary supplementation, and honest advertising, policies intended to ameliorate the deleterious impacts of poverty have also focused on food and nutrition. Prompted by both the recognition of widespread malnutrition and undernourishment among America's poor and the need to support farming in period of surplus, the middle decades of the twentieth century saw widespread expansion of federal policies to provide food assistance to school children, low income households, pregnant women, the elderly, and others in need. Franklin Roosevelt's New Deal greatly expanded the purpose of America's federal government, adopting measures to support beleaguered farmers while increasing food access to hungry Americans through food stamps and school lunches. Many of these programs were suspended with the start of WWII, as food supplies were redeployed to the military and Depression-era rates of unemployment evaporated. But the federal government's important role in ameliorating food insecurity was cemented through Lyndon Johnson's War on Poverty. Food stamps had reemerged as a pilot program in 1961 but, during the Johnson years, became a permanent entitlement program with the Food Stamp Act of 1964. The Child Nutrition Act of 1966 authorized free and low-cost milk and free and low-cost breakfast programs. In 1968, federal support was initiated for a summer foods program. These programs and policies focused primarily on increased consumption and ameliorating conditions of poverty rather than on dietary health or food choices per se. Their success can be seen in the reduced incidence of both poverty and hunger in the immediate years that followed (Brown and Allen 1988; Morrill 2015).

The many remarkable successes in food policy that characterized the late nineteenth and twentieth centuries required little need for behavioral change at the individual level. Effective public policies reduced food-borne illnesses, diseases of dietary insufficiency, and hunger without the need to change the way people purchased or consumed food. But now, addressing the link between food and health, as experienced in these early years of the twenty-first century, is even more complicated. Like other wicked problems, there is no single supplement, food-processing practice, or dietary change that will solve it. Addressing the rising levels of dietary-based health problems requires us to change human behavior, the very relationship between people and what they eat, and there is no easy way to accomplish this. Clinical approaches that rely on short-term one-on-one advice are too limited in scope and in scale; relatively few people receive such services, and without long-term support, most people who do receive such services for weight loss, for example, still regain lost weight over time (Hall and Kahan 2018). Yet while public policies have attempted to help ensure that people have access to more and safer food, relatively few policies, until recent years, have been focused on changing Americans' overall diet and general eating habits.

If we are to make meaningful inroads in the use of diet to reduce morbidity and mortality, we need to adopt a perspective on changing behaviors oriented toward populations; it must sit between the systems change of the last century and the clinical and individually oriented approaches of nutrition and health-care practice. In other words, we need to place individual decisions and choices within the context of a food environment that results from a host of policy decisions. Public policies aimed at reducing tobacco use provide an illustrative backdrop.

Dramatic reductions in smoking followed previously unimaginable policies aimed at changing the environment within which smoking occurs. Supplying smokers with information on smoking's health risks was not sufficient to change behavior, nor was smoke cessation counseling provided by well-minded clinicians. Rather, the rate of smoking was significantly reduced with the use of several important public policy levers, including taxes on cigarette purchases, bans on smoking in airplanes, restaurants, and workplaces, removal of subsidies to tobacco farmers, and restrictions on advertising combined with the public's education on the detrimental effects of smoking on health (Cummings 2002). As these policies were adopted, in varying order across different governmental units and jurisdictions (localities, states, and nations), cultural attitudes toward tobacco also began to shift. And as the culture shifted in its attitude toward tobacco, from the positive to the negative, governments adopted increasingly aggressive policies aimed at reducing its use. None of this was accomplished without a fight. Big Tobacco used an arsenal of tactics aimed at avoiding restrictions to its trade (Brownell and Warner 2009). But as the evidence mounted and norms began to shift, the courts supported the government's right to control the sale of tobacco in the name of the public's health.

Of course, tobacco and tobacco policy provide a less than perfect analogy for diet and food policy. Compared with diet, the message on tobacco is clear and easy: there is no safe level of smoking. Successful policies that made smoking both more expensive and more difficult were not aimed at modifying smoking behaviors but eradicating them. Further, in many cases, the legal argument for government intervention hinged on the dangers of second-hand smoke (that is, the deleterious impact of the smoker's behavior on the non-smoker), as well as on the importance of protecting children from becoming addicted to smoking before they were able to make adult decisions.

Diet, however, is far more complex. Finding public policies that will help promote healthier diets will need to be more nuanced and will likely need to be even more multifaceted. Further, in a political system that relies on a free-market economy, the government will likely be more restricted in its approaches to eating behaviors. There is little direct impact of one's dietary choices on their neighbor's health. Evidence of dietary addictions is thin even as our tastes and preferences may be shaped in childhood. As with tobacco, however, the interplay between law and policy, on the one hand, and history, culture, and agricultural economics, on the other, is especially relevant to thinking about how food policies might be used to improve the healthfulness of the American diet.

We are living in a time of extensive experimentation in the realm of food policy. Governments and foundations are trying to shape and reshape food policies to increase the likelihood of improved diets and, in turn, improved health. Yet each of these policies has had only limited impact, at best, in addressing problems of poor dietary quality and obesity. In the rest of this chapter, I will explore three general areas of food policy activity: increased access to healthful retail food options, calorie labeling in restaurants and fast-food venues, and taxes on sugars and sugar-sweetened beverages. I will briefly discuss the range of policies within each category, the assumptions undergirding them, and the research evidence regarding their effectiveness. Most especially, I will consider how a food studies lens might help us improve these policies; how would policies be changed if we recognized the importance of tradition and beauty, agriculture and waste disposal to our dietary choices? While public policy is interdisciplinary in approach, incorporating theories and methods of economics, politics, sociology, psychology, and statistics, as well as, more recently, psychology, issues of aesthetics, culture, history, and business are infrequently discussed. How might our approach to food policy be improved were this not the case?

How Food Policy Might be Enhanced with a Food Studies Lens: Three Case Examples

Policies to Improve Access to Healthier Foods in Food Deserts

Food deserts has become a commonly used phrase to capture the scarcity of retail food options, especially those offering healthy food, in poorer communities. In a world where supermarkets and big box stores are more likely to be opened and maintained in places with large enough populations and deep enough pockets, large-scale retailers have become increasingly scarce in both rural communities and impoverished neighborhoods in cities and suburbs, especially those with large concentrations of people of color and histories of discriminatory housing practices (Sadler, Bilal, and Furr-Holden 2021). The racialized aspect of food access has led some to adopt the phrase *food apartheid*. Since people living in locales with poor food access also have worse health outcomes than others and are less likely to consume recommended amounts of fruits and vegetables, many have concluded that the lack of access to nutritious food is the driver of these poor outcomes. Further, it has been assumed that if we used public policies (such as tax incentives) to motivate the siting of supermarkets in these food deserts or, alternatively, created other venues (such as greenmarkets and green carts) to sell fruits and vegetables in these communities, eating patterns would change. As it turns out, the very notion of food deserts may not be exactly right, and further, while policies can successfully increase food outlets in these communities, desired changes in diets do not necessarily result.

Geography does not, by itself, define access. While people may not live within walking distance of a well-stocked supermarket, this presents a problem only when those households lack a car or another easy form of transportation. The construct of a food desert makes sense only when the distance to a food retailer is not easily surmounted. As it turns out, this is a relatively rare situation in the United States; approximately 2 percent of American households live more than one mile from a supermarket and do not own a car (Rhone et al. 2019). Poor geographic access to food retailers is most salient in rural communities (Rhone et al. 2019). Further, when supermarkets have been incentivized, through policies like tax rebates, to locate into areas without such options, local residents do not necessarily choose to change their shopping patterns (Cummins, Flint, and Matthews 2014; Dubowitz et al. 2015a; Ghosh-Dastidara et al. 2017; Elbel et al. 2017). And even if they do, shopping in a supermarket, with its plethora of snack food, soda, and other manufactured food products, does not, in and of itself, change what a family buys and eats. Indeed, supermarkets are a major source of "junk food" purchases (Vaughan et al. 2017). New and improved supermarkets seem more likely to improve people's attitudes toward their neighborhoods and even increase property values than to change dietary behaviors (Caceres and Geoghegan 2017; Dubowitz et al. 2015b).

Creating other opportunities for the purchase of fruits and vegetables is also challenging. The most prominent examples are focused primarily on urban areas. Greenmarkets, with their emphasis on local produce, have proven to be a mixed blessing for local farmers; they expand their markets but also are labor intensive and lack the consistency of sales at scale. Further, in many parts of the United States, climate limits the growing season and thus their impact on what can be sold throughout the cold weather seasons. Greenmarkets, like supermarkets, have, been shown to be of broader economic value to the community and pleasing to neighborhood residents. They have become a source of educational information about food and cooking. But there is thin evidence that the simple presence of a greenmarket in a neighborhood is a significant driver in changes to diet or health outcomes (McCormack et al. 2010).

Greencarts—mobile carts selling fruits and vegetables to people on their way to work, school, or shopping—have also been tried by New York City to increase access to healthful food, especially in neighborhoods where such access has been more limited. This policy aims to create small business opportunities for the vendors at the same time as it aims to improve household diets. Some success has been found in regard to increases in the purchase of fresh fruits and vegetables (Farley et al. 2015).

Using a food studies lens, we should not be surprised by the limited success of these policies to improve diets and health through improved access to food retail spaces. History reminds us that supermarkets are a relatively recent and, perhaps, short-lived approach for food sales. Supermarkets emerged in the mid-twentieth century in response to the baby boom, suburbanization, and changing technology; supermarkets would make little sense without that era's larger kitchens, newly purchased refrigerators, and expanded use of automobiles. Prior to that, small grocers and specialized food shops (bakeries, butchers, and fishmongers) dominated the food landscape. Now we have seen the emergence of big box stores, as well as retail centers that sell clothing and electronics along with food. Food delivery services, an emerging substitute for supermarket shopping, became ever more central with the COVID-19 lockdowns. Recognizing these historical trends suggests that overemphasis on the siting of supermarkets may be misplaced. If our lives are now lived differently from the mid-twentieth century, shouldn't we expect our approach to grocery shopping to be different as well? How and where we purchase food is shaped by a wide range of current cultural norms and practices.

Giving more thought to the role of supermarkets and emerging retail alternatives seems smart as we move forward with policies to improve food access. Similarly, while the automobile has been important to retail food access in recent decades, pre-pandemic shifts among younger Americans away from automobile ownership suggest that we may need to consider policies that find other means to connect households to their food. With these historical and cultural trends in view, policies can be made to think forward rather than look backward.

Further, while greenmarkets have strengthened the ties between cities and their agricultural outskirts, the effectiveness of greenmarkets to sustain local agriculture or provide an ongoing source of healthful food has been limited. Certainly, greater emphasis on specific regional patterns for the growing and transportation of fruits and vegetables is needed. Additionally, finding ways to create more certain sales for these farmers requires thinking about the food system more broadly; supplementing the purchases of individual consumers with those of restaurants and institutional buyers creates a stronger economic base for local agriculture. Such solutions have been emerging but public policies aimed at expanding greenmarkets could do more to incorporate these ideas. Direct to consumer sales must recognize the commercial needs of local farmers if they are to succeed.

Greencarts, which build nicely off the tradition of street vendors in many older, American cities like New York, can serve as a worthwhile retail food supplement in those cities that have meaningful street traffic. But like greenmarkets, their effectiveness and sustainability also would benefit from a broader food systems perspective; for example, the recent ban on single-use plastic bags, an important step for the environment, will likely be problematic for these vendors, at least in the short run. From farming through disposal, policies aimed at improving food access need to consider how various retail options fit into the larger system.

Perhaps most importantly, the entire emphasis on food retail may be misplaced as the number of meals eaten out of the house has surpassed those eaten at home. Changing family structures, especially the role of women in the workplace and the rise of single-person households, and the associated shifts in cultural norms about how meals are prepared and where they are eaten, may constrain the value of these retail-focused public policies. Can one change dietary behavior through food retail when restaurants have become so dominant? Understanding this enormous shift in our eating practice requires far greater attention to our changing culture and societal expectations.

Calorie Labels in Fast-Food and Restaurant Outlets

Even as the notion of food deserts has received substantial attention in the world of food policy, the growth in restaurant-prepared meals has not gone unnoticed. "Food swamps" are those communities where unhealthful food options, especially in the form of fast-food outlets, are dense and dominant. As already noted, supermarket aisles are filled with many items that are decidedly less than healthful, and home cooking does not guarantee healthy eating. Even so, food prepared out of the home has been found to be more dense in calories, fats, and salt than that prepared at home (Lachat et al. 2012; Lin and Guthrie 2012). As Americans have become increasingly reliant on fast food and restaurants for their daily meals, policies to help people choose healthier options in those settings have also emerged.

Policies requiring calorie labels at fast-food establishments were rolled out first by several large cities and counties and then by states.

It has since become federal law in the United States under the Affordable Care Act, which expanded coverage to a wider array of eating establishments including sit-down restaurant chains. Undergirding calorie labeling policies is a set of assumptions about how the provision of information will encourage consumers to make different and better choices. What is perhaps surprising is how little evidence there is of the effectiveness of such labels. Indeed, few high-quality studies have found significant changes in purchases as a result of calorie labels alone, although it is worth noting that most such research has been conducted in fast-food and not sit-down restaurants (Bleich et al. 2017; Sinclair, Cooper, and Mansfield 2014).

Contrary to the assumptions undergirding these policies, people purchase meals at fast-food restaurants because they are fast and convenient (Rydell et al. 2008). They are not choosing such venues because they believe the food to be healthful, and many consumers never even notice the calorie labels, not to mention use the information provided by the labels (Breck et al. 2017). The broader context in which fast food is purchased does not well support the use of the calorie information, which requires attention to menu details and time for deliberation and reconsideration of options. In a world in which fast food is chosen because it is readily available and reliable and can be purchased and consumed during scarce free time, the mere provision of this information is unlikely to make a difference at scale.

As an alternative to calorie labels, some studies have experimented with more symbolic forms for sharing health information about menu options. For example, use of "red light, green light" symbols or check marks have been used to signal healthier and less healthy options, often with an emphasis on calorie density. Several countries are incorporating such an approach. For example, Chile introduced a "traffic light" labeling system aimed at reducing consumer confusion (Denecken 2018). Many in Europe have also adopted such a system (Jung-Mounib 2020). Symbols such as saltshakers have been tried to provide easier to use nutrition information to the public; New York City became the first city in the United States to require such symbolic information for high-sodium items on restaurant chain menus (NYC Health 2015). To what degree such visual or interpretive clues will be more effective in reshaping dietary choices remains a question, although it appears more promising than the posting of num-bers (Roy and Alassadi 2021; Sinclair, Cooper, and Mansfield 2014).

The shift from the use of numbers to one of colors and pictures fits nicely into the food studies framework. Relatively little attention was given to the aesthetics of the early calorie labels. While font size was written into the policy, the emphasis was on readability not on meaning or usability. While marketing executives have long thought about ad-vertising in terms of culture and beauty, the importance of these values to messaging was, essentially, neglected in developing the calorie label policies. Unlike colleagues in communications or cultural anthropology, I, as a student of health policy, was not exposed to semiotics; I did not think about the meaning or importance of symbols. Indeed, in present-ing research on the impact of calorie labels in my food policy class, l was challenged by a student whose work was in food marketing; it was he who crystallized for me that policies regarding calorie labels would have greatly benefited from the inclusion of the semiotic lens.

Additionally, while improving the information available to consum-ers is decidedly good, assuming that it, by itself, will change dietary behavior seems naive. If, for example, changes in family composition, the nature of work, and cultural expectations have led to a greater reli-ance on food that is fast, convenient, and reliable, greater emphasis on how policies might be used to change the food environment to meet these needs in a healthful way seems urgent. Recognizing how and why the food system has grown fast food to meet customer needs might allow us to craft policies to meet these needs in other manners. While the COVID-19 pandemic brought many people back to their kitchen, and although we may continue to see some additional information on home food preparation, the continued reliance on out-of-home options is likely to grow, especially as busy families return to in-person school and work.

At the same time, there is emerging evidence that calorie labels might have more impact on food industry decisions than consumer choices per se, as required labels appear to be changing product formulation (Grummon et al. 2021). It is a reminder that decisions in the private commercial sector can also be shaped by public policies. A food studies lens, which more readily embraces entrepreneurship and private sector endeavors, could be helpful in thinking about such policies.

Taxing Soda to Reduce Sugar Consumption

The emergence of soda taxes and, more broadly, sugar taxes signals a willingness to use economic tools to nudge individuals to make different dietary choices away from those products high in sugar-based calories. Such taxes have been adopted at the national level in countries outside of the United States; for example, in 2014, Mexico became the first country in the Americas to introduce a tax on sugar sweetened beverages (Vilar-Comte 2018). At the same time, numerous localities in the United States have imposed such taxes and they are under consideration in several states at the time of this writing (Boesen 2021). The use of taxes to curtail purchases of tobacco and alcohol has been demonstrated to be effective (Chisholm 2018; Goel and Nelson 2006; Wright, Smith, and Hellowell 2017). Sugar taxes aim to repeat this success.

Added sugar, however, is ubiquitous within processed foods; it is not, like tobacco or alcohol, generally purchased or consumed as a separate and distinct product. And while there is strong evidence that "too much" added sugar is a health problem, there is far less evidence that some is problematic. Indeed, small amounts of added sugar can make an otherwise healthful product more palatable. As a result, food policies efforts have focused more narrowly on soda rather than sugar taxes. Sugar-sweetened beverages, such as soda, share some similarities with tobacco in that it has no health benefit and, at least in large enough quantities, clear health risk.

As with tobacco in the mid-twentieth century, sodas are enjoyed by many and have been viewed, until recently, with limited concern by policymakers and the general public. There is, in a sense, no shame in ordering pop or soda with one's meal. Products like Coca-Cola, like the well-known cigarette brands of prior decades, are widely recognized symbols of pleasure in American society. Further, just as with Big Tobacco, the beverage industry is a formidable opponent of restrictive legislation; like with tobacco, the soda industry has engaged in aggressive lobbying against these policies while also adopting some limited self-imposed restrictions aimed at keeping the government at bay (Nestle 2015). Such corporate tactics have not been limited to the United States (Vilar-Compte 2018). Given the similarities and given the success of tobacco taxes in reducing smoking, taxes are to many in the world of health policy a potentially effective strategy for reducing soda consumption.

At the same time, reducing tobacco consumption required a far wider set of policy changes than just taxation. Little by little, measures were put in place at all levels of government to reduce advertising, limit how and where cigarettes could be purchased (for example, once ubiquitous vending machines were outlawed), and greatly restrict the places where people could smoke. Taxation has succeeded within this larger context and as complementary public education campaigns stressing the dangers of smoking reinforced the main message.

Can sugar-sweetened beverage taxes be as effective as those on tobacco? First, at this point in time, the taxes are far smaller than those imposed on tobacco. Early research indicates that taxes must be large enough to be "felt" if behaviors are to be changed; research suggests a 20 percent tax threshold (Wright, Smith, and Hellowell 2017). But of equal importance, we are unlikely to see the full array of policies aimed at curbing soda sales as those that were aimed at tobacco sales. Culturally, tobacco was long understood as an addictive product that was inappropriate for youngsters; that has not been the case for soda. Unlike tobacco, sugar-sweetened beverages are not "adults only." Much of the legislation curbing tobacco sales was sold, politically and legally, as protecting children. Further, the dangers of secondhand smoke were an important element in defending anti-tobacco legislation against legal arguments; for example, tobacco bans in airplanes and restaurants rested on the harm done to the health of flight attendants and restaurant workers. No such secondary harm can be claimed for sugar-sweetened beverages. For these reasons, it will be politically and legally difficult to constrain sales of sodas, given industry pushback and resources (Nestle 2015). Efforts in NYC, for example, to curb soda consumption by limiting the size of drinks in fast-food settings were thwarted by the courts. In the decision, the court noted that they did not view sugar-sweetened beverages as "inherently harmful," even as research has repeatedly demonstrated a deleterious effect on health and longevity (Malik et al. 2019; Malik et al. 2010).

At the same time, unlike with tobacco, the beverage industry has been able to capitalize on the availability of marketable substitutes in reducing sales of sugar-sweetened beverages. In some cases, "diet" sodas are not taxed, allowing soda manufacturers to encourage consumers to switch away from sugar-sweetened drinks to those with sugar substitutes. Even more dramatically, these companies have substantially increased their sales of bottled waters; the bottom line stays intact, even if soda sales plummet.

Using a food studies lens to consider the likely effects of a soda tax would allow us to consider likely impacts in a more nuanced way and would perhaps provide a better sense of complementary approaches to reducing soda consumption. A food studies lens would encourage us to see that not all products and purchases are the same. While a tax might be the solution for one good, it is not necessarily the right approach for another. This is not to argue against the potential benefit of a soda tax but rather to encourage greater attention to how sugar-sweetened beverages fit into a style of eating. What is the meaning of these drinks? Why are people choosing them? What would allow for the kind of cultural shift away from them just as we did for tobacco, given that similarly restrictive policies are not likely to be adopted? Ethnography and other qualitative research methods, less frequently used in health policy than in other areas of food studies, might bring more light to our understanding of beverage choices. A food studies lens would encourage more attention to the pleasure of the drink; a small tax alone is likely not sufficient for people to give up such a pleasure. Further, if through these taxes we are encouraging a shift away from soda to bottled waters, what are the implications for the environment? Will this emphasis on bottled water move people away from tap water and encourage even greater use of plastic waste?

Bringing It Together

As all of this policy activity suggests, I am far from alone in bringing public policy experience, skills, and training to the study of food policy and health. I would argue, however, that being situated in a program in food studies makes me somewhat unusual. Rather than being surrounded by similarly trained scholars in public policy or similarly focused researchers in public health, I have been working among colleagues who focus on food from the perspective of culture, history, and agricultural economics. In trying to address the real-world problems associated with diet and health, I have been pushed by my colleagues and my students to consider the importance of aesthetics, values, and the larger context of the food system, from agricultural production through waste disposal, to the likely effectiveness of government food policies. Even as the field of food studies grows and morphs, its view of the food system as an interrelated whole and its encouragement of inter-disciplinary engagement has required me to open my work to new ideas and new perspectives. Hopefully, teams of scholars with a more diverse set of backgrounds, perspectives, and assumptions will allow for more effective policy making.

REFERENCES

Aschemann-Witzel, Jessica, Frederico J. A. Perez-Cueto, Barbara Niedzwiedzka, Wim Verbeke, and Tino Bech-Larsen. 2012. "Lessons for Public Health Campaigns from Analysing Commercial Food Marketing Success Factors: A Case Study." *BMC Public Health* 12, no. 139 (February 21). https://doi.org/10.1186/1471-2458-12-139.

Bleich, Sara N., Christina D. Economos, Marie L. Spiker, Kelsey A. Vercammen, Eric M. VanEpps, Jason P. Block, Brian Elbel, Mary Story, and Christina A. Roberto. 2017. "A Systematic Review of Calorie Labeling and Modified Calorie Labeling Interventions: Impact on Consumer and Restaurant Behavior." *Obesity* 25 (12): 2018–44. doi: 10.1002/oby.21940.

Boesen, Ulrik. 2021. "Sugar Taxes Back on the Menu." *Tax Foundation*, February 18. https://taxfoundation.org.

Breck, Andrew, Tod Mijanovich, Beth C. Weitzman, and Brin Elbel. 2017. "The Current Limits of Calorie Labeling and the Potential for Population Health Impact." *Journal of Public Policy & Marketing* 36:2172–79.

Brown, Larry J., and Deborah Allen. 1988. "Hunger in America." *Annual Review of Public Health* 9:503–26.

Brownell, Kelly D., and Kenneth E. Warner. 2009. "The Perils of Ignoring History: Big Tobacco Played Dirty and Millions Died. How Similar Is Big Food?" *Milbank Quarterly* 87:259–94. https://doi.org/10.1111/j.1468-0009.2009.00555.x.

Buzby, Jean. 2006. "Possible Implications for U.S. Agriculture from Adoption of Select Dietary Guidelines." United States Department of Agriculture Economic Research Report Number 31. https://www.ers.usda.gov.

Caceres, Belkis Cerrato, and Jacqueline Geoghegan. 2017. "Effects of New Grocery Store Development on Inner-City Neighborhood Residential Prices." *Agricultural and Resource Economics Review* 46 (1): 87–102. doi:10.1017/age.2016.29.

Centers for Disease Control and Prevention (CDC). 1998. "Achievements in Public Health, 1900–1999: Safer and Healthier Foods." *Morbidity and Mortality Weekly Report* 48, no. 40 (October 15): 905–913. https://www.cdc.gov.

Centers for Medicare and Medicaid Services. n.d. *NEH Fact Sheet*. https://www.cms .gov/. Accessed January 20, 2022.

Chisholm, Dan, Daniela Moro, Melanie Bertram, Carel Pretorius, Gerrit Gmel, Kevin Shield, and Jürgen Rehm. 2018. "Are the 'Best Buys' for Alcohol Control Still Valid? An Update on the Comparative Cost-Effectiveness of Alcohol Control Strategies at the Global Level." *Journal of Studies on Alcohol and Drugs* 79:514. doi: 10.15288 /jsad.2018.79.514.

Cummings, K. Michael. 2002. "Programs and Policies to Discourage the Use of Tobacco Products." *Oncogene* 21:7349–64. https://doi.org/10.1038/sj.onc.1205810.

Cummins, Steven, Ellen Flint, and Stephen A. Matthews. 2014. "New Neighborhood Store Increased Awareness of Food Access but Did Not Alter Dietary Habits or Obesity." *Health Affairs* 33:283–91.

Denecken A. A. 2018. "Development and Implementation Processes of the Food Labeling and Advertising Law in Chile." Global Delivery Initiative, World Bank Group. https://effectivecooperation.org/system/files/2021-06/GDI%20Case%20Study%20 -%20Food%20Labeling%20and%20Advertising%20Law%20in%20Chile.pdf.

Dubowitz, Tamara, Madhumita Ghosh-Dastidar, Deborah A. Cohen, Robin Beckman, Elizabeth D. Steiner, Gerald P. Hunter, Karen R. Flórez, et al. 2015a. "Diet and Perceptions Change with Supermarket Introduction in a Food Desert, but Not Because of Supermarket Use." *Health Affairs* 34 (11): 1858–68. https://doi.org/10.1377/hlthaff .2015.0667.

———. 2015b. "A New Supermarket in a Food Desert: Is Better Health in Store?" Santa Monica, CA: RAND Corporation. https://www.rand.org/.

Elbel, Brian, Tod Mijanovich, Kamila Kiszko, Courtney Abrams, Jonathan Cantor, and L. Beth Dixon. 2017. "The Introduction of a Supermarket via Tax-Credits in a Low-Income Area." *American Journal of Health Promotion* 31 (1): 59–66. doi: 10.4278 /ajhp.150217-QUAN-733.

Farley, Shannon M., Rachel Sacks, Rachel Dannefer, Michael Johns, Margaret Leggat, Sungwoo Lim, Kevin Konty, and Cathy Nonas. 2015. "Evaluation of the New York City Green Carts Program." *AIMS Public Health* 2 (4): 906–18. doi:10.3934 /publichealth.2015.4.906.

Ghosh-Dastidara, Madhumita, Gerald Hunter, Rebecca L. Collins, Shannon N. Zenk, Steven Cummins, Robin Beckman, Alvin K. Nugroho, Jennifer C. Sloan, La'Vette Wagnerand, and Tamara Dubowitz. 2017. "Does Opening a Supermarket in a Food Desert Change the Food Environment?" *Health and Place* 46:249–56. doi:10.1016/j .healthplace.2017.06.002.

Goel, Rajeev K., and Michael A. Nelson. 2006. "The Effectiveness of Anti-Smoking Legislation: A Review." *Journal of Economic Surveys* 20, no. 3 (July): 325–55. https:// doi.org/10.1111/j.0950-0804.2006.00282.x.

Grummon, Anna H., Joshua Petimar, Fang Zhang, Anjali Rao, Steven L. Gortmaker, Eric B. Rimm, and Sara N. Bleich, et al. 2021. "Calorie Labeling and Product Reformulation: A Longitudinal Analysis of Supermarket-Prepared Foods." *American Journal of Preventative Medicine* 61, no. 3 (September): 377–85. doi: 10.1016/j.amepre.2021.03.013.

Hajar, Rachel. 2016. "Framingham Contribution to Cardiovascular Disease." *Heart Views* 17, no. 2 (April–June): 78–81. https://doi.org/10.4103/1995-705X.185130.

Hall, Kevin D., and Scott Kahan. 2018. "Maintenance of Lost Weight and Long-Term Management of Obesity." *Medical Clinics of North America* 102, no. 1 (January): 183–97. doi: 10.1016/j.mcna.2017.08.012.

Jung-Mounib, Monika. 2020. "Food Labelling System, Nutri-Score, Gains Momentum in Europe." *Quality Assurance and Food Safety*, April 3. https://www.qualityassurance mag.com.

Lachat, C., E. Nago, R. Verstraeten, D. Roberfroid, J. Van Camp, and P. Kolsteren. 2012. "Eating out of Home and Its Association with Dietary Intake: A Systematic Review of the Evidence." *Obesity Reviews* 13, no. 4 (April): 329–46. https://doi. org/10.1111/j.1467-789X.2011.00953.x.

Lin, Biing Hwan, and Joanne Guthrie. 2012. "Nutritional Quality of Food Prepared at Home and Away From Home, 1977–2008." USDA Economic Research Service Economic Information Bulletin 105. Washington, DC: United States Department of Agriculture.

Loef, Martin, and Harald Walach. 2012. "The Combined Effects of Healthy Lifestyle Behaviors on All Cause Mortality: A Systematic Review and Meta-Analysis." *Preventive Medicine* 55, no. 3 (September): 163–70. doi:10.1016/j.ypmed.2012.06.017.

Malik, Vasanti S., Yanping Li, An Pan, Lawrence De Koning, Eva Schernhamme, Walter C. Willett, and Frank B Hu. 2019. "Long-Term Consumption of Sugar-Sweetened and Artificially Sweetened Beverages and Risk of Mortality in US Adults." *Circulation*, 139, no. 18 (April): 2113–215. doi: 10.1161/CIRCULATIONAHA .118.037401.

Malik, Vasanti S., Barry M. Popkin, George A. Bray, Jean-Pierre Després, and Frank B. Hu. 2010. "Sugar-Sweetened Beverages, Obesity, Type 2 Diabetes Mellitus, and Cardiovascular Disease Risk." *Circulation* 121, no. 11 (March 23): 1356–64 doi .org/10.1161/CIRCULATIONAHA.109.876185.

McCormack, Lacey Arneson, Melissa Nelson Laska, Nicole I. Larson, and Mary Story. 2010. "Review of the Nutritional Implications of Farmers' Markets and Community Gardens: A Call for Evaluation and Research Efforts. *Journal of the American Dietetic Association* 110, no. 3 (March 10): 399–408. doi: 10.1016/j.jada.2009.11.023.

Morrill, Richard. 2015. "50 Years of US Poverty: 1960 to 2010." *Newgeography*, February 19. http://www.newgeography.

Neff, Roni A., Kathleen Merrrigan, and David Wallinga. 2015. "A Food Systems Approach to Healthy Food and Agriculture." *Health Affairs*, 34, no. 11 (November): 1908–15. doi: 10.1377/hlthaff.2015.0926.

Nestle, Marion. 2002. *Food Politics*. Berkeley: University of California Press.

———. 2015. *Soda Politics: Taking on Big Soda (and Winning)*. Berkeley: University of California Press.

New York City (NYC) Health. 2015. "Sodium Initiatives." https://www1.nyc.gov.

New York State Health Foundation. n.d. "Healthy Food, Healthy Lives." https:// nyshealthfoundation.org/.

Rhone, Alana, Michele Ver Ploeg, Ryan Williams, and Vince Breneman. 2019. "Understanding Low-Income and Low-Access Census Tracts across the Nation:

Subnational and Subpopulation Estimates of Access to Healthy Food." USDA Economic Research Service, Economic Information Bulletin Number 209. Washington, DC: United Sates Department of Agriculture.

Robert Wood Johnson Foundation (RWJF) n.d. Accessed July 6, 2023. https://www.rwjf.org.

Roy, Rajshri, and Deema Alassadi. 2021. "Does Labelling of Healthy Foods on Menus Using Symbols Promote Better Choices at the Point-of-Purchase?" *Public Health Nutrition*, 24 (4): 746–54. doi:10.1017/S1368980020002840.

Rydell, Sarah A., Lisa J. Harnack, J. Michael Oakes, Mary Story, Robert W. Jeffrey, and Simone A. French. 2008. "Why Eat at Fast-Food Restaurants: Reported Reasons among Frequent Consumers." *Journal of the American Dietetic Association* 108 (12), 2066–70. doi: 10.1016/j.jada.2008.09.008.

Sadler, Richard C., Usama Bilal, and C. Debra Furr-Holden. 2021. "Linking Historical Discriminatory Housing Patterns to the Contemporary Food Environment in Baltimore." *Spatial and Spatio-temporal Epidemiology*, 36. https://doi.org/10.1016/j.sste.2020.100387.

Sinclair, Susan E., Marcia Cooper, and Elizabeth D. Mansfield. 2014. "The Influence of Menu Labeling on Calories Selected or Consumed: A Systematic Review and Meta-Analysis." *Journal of the Academy of Nutrition and Dietetics* 114, no. 9 (September): 1375–88. https://doi.org/10.1016/j.jand.2014.05.014.

Social Security Administration. n.d. "Social Security History." Accessed January 20 2022. https://www.ssa.gov/history/ottob.html.

United States Food and Drug Administration (USFDA). 2018. "Changes in Science, Law and Regulatory Authorities." January 31. https://www.fda.gov.

Vaughan, Christine, Deborah A. Cohen, Madhumita Ghosh-Dastidar, Gerald P; Hunter, and Tamar Dubowitz. 2017. "Where Do Food Desert Residents Buy Most of Their Junk Food? Supermarkets." *Public Health Nutrition*, 20, no. 14 (October): 2608–16. doi:10.1017/S136898001600269X.

Vilar-Compte, Mireya. 2018. "Using Sugar-Sweetened Beverages Taxes and Advertising Regulations to Combat Obesity in Mexico." World Bank Group, Global Delivery Initiative. https://effectivecooperation.org.

Wright, Alex, Katherine E. Smith, and Mark Hellowell. 2017. "Policy Lessons from Health Taxes: A Systematic Review of Empirical Studies." *BMC Public Health* 17 (1): 583. https://doi.org/10.1186/s12889-017-4497-z.

6

Applied Nutrition

Experiencing Well-Being beyond Nutrients

LISA SASSON

My professional career has been devoted to understanding how nutrition and healthy lifestyle habits can improve the quality of people's lives. I was drawn to the science of nutrition because of my passion for food, the role food plays in one's culture, and because of my fascination with the relationship of nutrients to disease development and prevention.

I have always had a deep-rooted love for food. My mother was a great cook, and growing up, the kitchen was the centerpiece of our home. My fondest childhood food memories are of my mother preparing dishes like Swiss steak, roast chicken, fried onions with mushrooms and barley, chicken noodle soup, and noodle pudding. I would watch with amazement as my mother, without using a cookbook, would fuse ingredients and make a delicious meal. The house was always filled with wonderful aromas that to this day bring back great food memories. For this reason, it was important to me that my children were exposed to and participated in cooking so they, too, would have wonderful food memories.

My interest in food expanded when I took my first trip, as a teenager, backpacking through Europe. I vividly recall tasting my first Greek salad in Athens. The tomatoes, cucumbers, feta cheese, and olive oil were delicious and tasted nothing like the tomatoes and cucumbers back in Queens, New York. Incomprehensible to today's generation of students, most of us at that time did not have exposure to food products and cuisines from around the world. I will never forget that first time I tried olive oil; the depth of flavor and attachment to the earth shaped my love for Mediterranean cuisine to this day. As I traveled around Europe, I shared meals with fellow backpackers from all over the world, expanding my palate and my curiosity. This experience cemented what would be a lifelong commitment to food and food cultures. As a nutritionist in the academy, I took with me this fascination with food and combined it with a desire to help people improve their quality of life. In this light, I have always seen nutrition and food studies as holistic, as crossing the boundaries of health and culture, environment and social justice.

Hence, this chapter explores how an interdisciplinary, experiential approach to nutrition can enrich the learning, relationships, and knowledge of students and can create a more collaborative future where dietitians, scholars, and other food professionals can work together. I will share a few examples of courses and projects I was able to create because the nutrition program at NYU is part of the larger Department of Nutrition and Food Studies (NFS) that includes culture, human development, and the psychological and sociological aspects of food. These include the Body Project, the Iron Chef Dysphagia Competition, and Global Study Abroad courses.

Food is a great unifier, as all humans and animals need to eat. Traditionally, a nutrition curriculum focuses on how food is digested, absorbed, and turned into energy in the body, how hormones regulate bodily processes, and what diets to recommend according to medical conditions to promote health. As a result, registered dietitians and nutrition graduate students are well versed in the science of food and nutrition and disease prevention and management. However, the reason people choose the foods they eat goes beyond daily requirements. What is often lacking in nutrition curricula is the focus on food as more than just sustenance for the body; food provides cultural significance and carries us throughout our lives as we age and grow. Food connects us to our ancestors and family. Food sits at the center of questions of social and racial equity. Food can be the source of both positive and negative psychological attachments to our body. And the list goes on. Being part of a food studies program has enhanced our nutrition curriculum to go beyond just the nutrient value of food and to see it for the greater force that it is.

Nutrition programs across the country can often be prescriptive, allowing little room for deviation from the rules. Dietetic programs follow science-heavy courses in a regimented order, with students taking the same classes and leaving with the same takeaways as the students before them. Until a few decades ago, most dietitians were thought of as "food service personnel" because historically, dietitians spent most of their time working with the kitchen staff to provide the appropriate medical meal or the right meal consistency (Barber 1959; USOPM 1980). Although a career in nutrition can be diverse, many programs, and the students who attend them, are not. Dietetic students are predominantly white, female, and from a higher socioeconomic status (there are concerted efforts to change this), but the clients and patients these future dietitians will be seeing are diverse, not so uniformly gendered, raced, or classed. In most nutrition programs, students are taught to focus on nutrients in their most basic components, but people are not going to the grocery store to shop for nutrients; they are shopping for whole foods, based on reasons such as culture, taste, income, education, cooking skills, and family habits.

Body Image Project

Food is more than just what we eat; it also affects how we view ourselves and those around us. Food consumption is often linked to self-worth and body image. Food offers an element of control; a restrictive eater may not be able to control the events around them but can control the content and quantity of what they consume. We often hear people refer to their daily food consumption as good or bad. Yet this binary leaves no room for the multitude of joy, pain, satisfaction, and sorrow that food may contain.

To connect students with the belief that food is more than just nutrients, when I was the director of the NYU dietetic internship, I challenged students to look further into their dietary consumption, beliefs, and feelings about food and to understand issues related to body image. In an anonymous exercise, students in our dietetic internship class were instructed to reflect on the role food has played in their lives. They were tasked with discussing their earliest memories of their body image, how others influence the way they see themselves, and what eating means to them. For many, that was the first time they put these thoughts and feelings on paper. We have students who wrote pages that contained years of buried emotions surrounding their relationship with food. Students found that assignment helpful and often cathartic and came back even years later to discuss how this exercise was the first time they had ever explored these thoughts and feelings. Here is what some of them had to say:

> Thank you for opening up a discussion that seems to be taboo in the dietetics curriculum. My past experiences related to food will allow me to better understand and connect with my clients.

> Having a better understanding of my complicated relationship with food and my body will make me a more compassionate counselor.

> This assignment was not easy for me to do, but it was so important. It was painful to think back to my childhood and how I struggled with my weight and food binging. I will use my past experiences to be a more empathetic nutrition counselor.

> I never experienced body weight or food issues but the struggles some of my classmates shared were eye opening. This project will make me a better listener and educator.

> I want to thank the students who were brave enough to share their past and current food and body image issues. I always felt so alone with my food and body weight thoughts. It was liberating to know my classmates also have struggled with these issues.

By exploring these beliefs, students have a better understanding about themselves and others to become more effective nutrition educators or counselors (Friedman 2008). The field of nutrition is one in which the primary focus is to help others; our curriculum incorporates counseling and psychology classes to foster these skills in our students. However, many nutrition and dietetic curricula do not touch on how a student's relationship to both food and their own body image can influence their interactions with clients and patients in their practice. Research has demonstrated that altered relationships to food may be a driver in why students elect to study dietetics in the first place. One paper notes "one-third of dietetics students are motivated to enter the field by personal experiences (self or friends) with obesity or eating disorders" (Houston, Bassler, and Anderson 2009).

A Need for a Transdisciplinary Approach:
Iron Chef Dysphagia Challenge

Being in a program that emphasizes culture and human behavior allowed me to create and co-teach the class An Interdisciplinary Case-Based Management of Dysphagia. This multidisciplinary class is focused on patient care in terms not only of medicine, nutrition therapy, and food safety but also of the culture of the patient and the happiness, memories, and sense of identity that food can bring.

Dysphagia, or difficulty with swallowing, can occur from a number of conditions such as head and neck cancer, dementia, Parkinson's disease, stroke, and traumatic brain injury. Patients often refuse to drink or eat, eat less, or are noncompliant with the diet. Dysphagia is particularly challenging because quite a lot of the food and beverage of the diet can be unappealing, leading to malnutrition, dehydration, and aspiration pneumonia with significant health-care expenditure and reduced health-care outcome.

The management of dysphagia requires an interdisciplinary approach, but practitioners from different disciplines view eating and nutrition through their own discipline-specific lenses (Heiss, Goldberg, and Dzarnoski 2010). For example, speech-language pathologists are concerned with anatomical and physiological aspects of swallowing for the diagnosis of dysphagia and make recommendations regarding food consistency for safe swallowing. Nutritionists are responsible for making sure that nutrition and hydration needs of the patient are met and may add nutritional supplements. Physicians add their own cocktail of drugs. The patient and family members are left to carry out the myriad recommendations to the best of their understanding with a lot being lost in translation.

The goal of the treatment of dysphagia is to enable patients to eat appealing, culturally appropriate, nutritious meals that fulfill their physical, emotional, and psychosocial needs (Winkler 2009). In this course that I coteach with a speech pathologist, nutrition students, speech language pathology students, and medical residents are brought together to provide care to a patient with a swallowing difficulty and create a therapeutic menu for them with respect to their culture, age, medical condition, and background. Texture-modified diets can be tough for patients to eat as they can be visually unappealing and make an already difficult diagnosis more challenging. This course encourages students to circumvent these barriers and work together to provide patients with appropriate meals they can actually enjoy (Heiss, Goldberg, and Dzarnoski 2010).

The course combines an academic and a hands-on component. Students compete in a timed cooking competition to prepare texturally, nutritional, tasty, eye-appealing, and culturally appropriate foods for their case study patient. They also collaborate to create a complete medical care plan and present their case study patient to the class and medical residents and at the NYU Langone Medical Center. A case study may be about a teenager with a traumatic brain injury from a car accident, for example, or an older adult who had a stroke, or a person who has dementia. The teams review barium swallows for their respective cases to measure the degree of difficulty their patients had when swallowing foods and liquids, and then they determine the consistency of their foods and beverages. On the final day of the class is the Iron Chef Dysphagia Contest. The teams have two hours in the kitchen to prepare a meal and beverage for their case study patient and will be judged by the following criteria: medical, safety, health, culture, and their patient's personal food preferences. The challenge is to create an appetizing and eye-appealing meal. This is no small task.

The six panel judges usually include a physiatrist, nutritionist, speech language pathologist, celebrity chef, food writer, and restaurateur who deliberate over the five dishes and beverages and decide which team is the Dysphagia Iron Chef winner. Quite often, the winning team had to create the most challenging diet—all pureed. One year, the winning dish was curried soup prepared for an older patient from India who had Alzheimer's disease. The team creatively topped the spicy soup with whipped chickpea mousse topping and a colorful layered pureed vegetable soufflé that brought an aesthetic quality to the dishes.

While this course is fun and the competition brings levity to the experience, students find that working across the aisle with other disciplines and learning to focus on patients on a broader scale affect the way they will practice in their future careers. Even the medical students and residents commented that this course influences their practice, with one chief resident saying he entirely "rethought" the way he would look at food going forward.

At the core of this course and others like it is the critical notion that food is one of the greatest sources of pleasure and joy. The aroma of a family meal may bring back a spark of a memory for a patient with de- mentia or a patient in hospice care. Providing a patient with a favorite meal allows the family and caregivers to take part of the patient's care and provides them with a way to express their love and care. Loved ones are often left out of the conversation when it comes to patient care, and this course reminds students that it is important to take care of caregiv- ers and families as well as patients. Patients whose full lives are included in their care benefit more than those that are just viewed as their disease or their symptoms. Food is a connector; it allows us to comfort, nour- ish, and nurture, and it might be the last love we can give to express how we feel. It is easier in medicine to deal with objective measures and facts, but once you start to probe and think of subjective information about patients, it becomes more personal and allows us to focus on what makes us uniquely human.

Study abroad Courses

NYU's NFS Department Global Study Abroad program offers students the opportunity to weave the cultural, spiritual, and social significance of food into their coursework. For so long, the discourse on healthful eating has focused on calorie restriction and eating less rather than savoring and enjoying good quality food. Most nutrition programs do not emphasize the importance of students' enjoying food and cooking, of having a passion for food. If a student is not a food lover, it may not be important to them how a food looks or tastes for their patient as long as the food is healthy and protects them against disease. But if a food is not tasty, eye appealing, and culturally appropriate, then it really does not matter how nutritious it is, since most people will not eat it (Contento 2011; European Food Information Council 2006).

New York University, nestled within the global city of New York, af- fords its students countless opportunities to explore the world and study the people and the culture that makes every corner of the globe unique. The NFS Department particularly encourages students to take their studies abroad and put what they have been learning into practice (more on the travel courses in the final chapter). With the privilege of traveling comes the invaluable experiences of not only learning about other cultures but also learning about oneself. Our global nutrition and food studies courses allow students of all disciplines to travel to countries and immerse themselves in the food and culture of those who reside there. Our global courses focus on food and culture, the joys of preparing and sharing meals, and the quality of the ingredients versus the obsession with their perceived health or caloric content. The experiential component strengthens these courses, as students are able to visit food markets and food producers, meet with farmers, participate in culinary classes, and sit down to share meals with their classmates. We have found that when people understand the value of sharing a meal, eating whole foods can lead to less obsession and better appreciation of food as something that not only sustains us but also provides us with some of the greatest joy of life.

Students who take this course find that it helps them grow both professionally and personally (Sasson, Black, and Dalton 2007). It opens their minds to perspectives and lifestyles that look nothing like their own. Food can be a point of entry that draws someone in; you may not speak someone's language or be able to partake in their cultural practices, but you may recognize, and love, their favorite dish and can share in that sense of belonging. This course allows for that feeling of belonging by transcending language and status and other barriers through food.

Food can also serve as a reminder of the history of a society and a culture, both how far it has come and how much it has remained unchanged. The risotto our students make in a cooking class, with roots in Italy dating back hundreds of years, provides them with more than just knowledge about the ingredients and preparation. Food is the medium through which older generations pass down their stories, their dreams for their futures, and their family traditions. The history of the foods we eat should not be overlooked when counseling clients or patients, although this is not often built into standard dietetics programs. Our nutrition program is strengthened by its being included in a department that focuses on all aspects of the foods we eat foods we have eaten, and the foods that will nourish our future.

Future Direction

Humans will continue spreading themselves to every corner of the globe and in doing so will continue creating new and innovative ways to consume food, produce it, and share in it. As we look toward the future of food, we cannot forget to focus on the larger impact our consumption is having on our resources and environment, as our current model is unsustainable. Nearly as important as the sociological, spiritual, and cultural impacts of food on society, the sustainability of the food we are eating and sharing should become part of a larger conversation for food studies students and nutrition students alike. To learn only about the biological value of the protein in the egg without touching on the production required to transport that egg from a factory farm to your local grocery store misses the larger picture.

We are teaching patients and families about the benefits of fruits and vegetables for their health but not about the environmental costs of having fresh fruits and vegetables available at their local grocery store in the middle of February. We continue to learn how many of our favorite foods—honey, avocados, wine, and chocolate—are in danger of not existing in a few short decades due to the environmental costs of their production, commodification, and consumption. How can we create learning environments where we extol the virtues of healthful foods without forgetting the real cost to the planet that produces them?

Food can be a political tool that can empower us as citizens of our countries. We can vote with our fork, we can eat with our conscience, and we can purchase with power. We can compost the foods we cook and bring reusable containers to restaurants, grocery stores, and dinner parties for leftovers. Dietetics has long been a profession that has focused on the microscopic effects of foods on bodies, but we continue to learn how impactful even one person's forkful is on our global food system. Meal prepping can be a great tool for healthful eating, but how much of the food we purchase or prepare is being wasted? What is the cost on communities that grow and labor to provide quinoa, kale, or any other "superfoods"? The field of dietetics, which historically focuses on the effects of foods on individuals, must continue to expand outward to include the effects of food on communities, cities, countries, and continents.

REFERENCES

Barber, Mary I., ed. 1959. *History of the American Dietetic Association, 1917–1959.* Philadelphia: J. B. Lippincott.

Contento, Isobel R., and Pamela A. Koch. 2011. *Nutrition Education: Linking Research, Theory and Practice.* 2nd ed. Burlington, MA: Jones & Bartlett.

European Food Information Council. 2016. "The Factors That Influence Our Food Choices." 2006. June 6. https://www.eufic.org.

Friedman, Richard A. 2008. "Have You Ever Been in Psychotherapy, Doctor?" *New York Times*, February 10. https://www.nytimes.com.

Heiss, Cynthia J., Lynette Ruth Goldberg, and Marisa Dzarnoski. 2010. "Registered Dietitians and Speech-Language Pathologists: An Important Partnership in Dysphagia Management." *Journal of the American Dietetic Association* 110, no. 9 (September): 1290, 1292–93. doi:10.1016/j.jada.2010.07.014.

Houston, Cheryl A., Eunice Bassler, and Jean Anderson. 2009. "Eating Disorders among Dietetic Students: An Educator's Dilemma." *Journal of American Dietetic Association* 108, no. 4 (April): 722–24. doi: 10.1016/j.jada.2008.01.048.

Sasson, Lisa, Jennifer Black, and Sharron Dalton. 2007. "Lessons Learned about Food-Related Attitudes and Behaviors from an Italian Study abroad Program." *Topics in Clinical Nutrition* 22, no. 4 (October): 357–66. doi:10.1097/01.TIN .0000308472.79813.7e.

United States Office of Personnel Management (USOPM). 1980. "Occupational Information." In *Position Classification Standard for Dietitian and Nutritionist Series, GS-0630*, 3–10. https://www.opm.gov.

Winkler, Marion. 2009. "Lenna Frances Cooper Memorial Lecture: Living with Enteral and Parenteral Nutrition: How Food and Eating Contribute to Quality of Life." 2010. *Journal of the American Dietetic Association* 110, no. 2 (February): 160–77. https://doi.org/10.1016/j.jada.2009.12.002.

7

Nutrition and Dietetics

Training Registered Dietitians within a Food Systems Framework

STEPHANIE ROGUS

Dietetics practice involves utilizing the nutrition care process to assess, diagnose, intervene, monitor, and evaluate the nutrition status of patients and clients (Gandy 2019). Food is an important component of dietetics; dietitians assess dietary intake and provide dietary recommendations for patients; they manage food operations in hospitals and school cafeterias; they implement federal, state, and local food and nutrition assistance programs. Traditionally, the field has focused on the health impacts of nutrient intake and dietary recommendations for individuals and populations but has failed to address the social, cultural, and environmental factors affecting food decisions, dietary quality beyond nutrient content, and the environmental, economic, and social impacts of the food system (Harmon et al. 2011; Wilkins 2009; Wilkins et al. 2010). Until recently, dietetics has remained largely unengaged with the food system.

The field of dietetics has been evolving over the past thirty years as calls for dietitians (RDNs) to take more active roles in the food system have emerged. The profession of dietetics may not have considered food systems as a relevant area of knowledge and expertise in the early 2000s, due in part to the narrow scope of the profession and traditional views on dietetics practice (Harmon et al. 2011, Wilkins 2009; Wilkins et al. 2010). However, the growth of interest in food system–related issues such as the widespread availability of nutrient-poor foods, the availability and quality of land and water for agricultural production, unhealthy dietary patterns, food safety, and food insecurity—often termed "wicked problems" because of their complexity in cause and consequence (Hamm 2009; Kreuter et al. 2004)—have drawn the attention of dietetics students and practitioners and fueled arguments for broadening the knowledge base of dietitians (Wegener 2018; Wilkins 2009).

This expanded view of the profession has been supported by academics, practitioners, and the Academy of Nutrition and Dietetics (the academy), which serves as the largest organization of nutrition and dietetics professionals in the United States. In accordance with this broadened view of the profession, it is important to consider how new and emerging disciplines, such as food studies, can be leveraged to meet the demands of dietetics students and practitioners.

The discipline of food studies seeks to understand the human relationship with food. It examines complex interconnections among food, culture, and society from perspectives of academics in the humanities, social sciences, and sciences (Almerico 2014; Miller and Deutsch 2009). It is more than simply an exploration of the production, preparation, and consumption of food, and it differs from other food-related fields, such as agricultural science, the culinary arts, nutrition, food science, agricultural economics, and gastronomy (Almerico 2014). In food studies, relationships between food and society are examined by scholars in several disciplines, including economics, nutrition, public health, public policy, education, sociology, history, and anthropology. It is a relatively new field that has taken root as an area of study at many universities, including New York University, where students generally focus on one of two tracks in food studies: food culture and food systems.

Food Systems in Dietetics

The study of food systems encompasses the "causes and consequences of [food] production and consumption" (Nestle and McIntosh 2010, 160). The food system includes methods of production, processing, distribution, retailing, and consumption (Neff, Merrigan, and Wallinga 2015). Although food systems within the field of food studies have been explored from various perspectives, including economic, social, biological, and behavioral, it was not until recently that dietitians began considering their role in understanding and intervening in food system issues that impact the health of populations and the environment (Nestle and McIntosh 2010).

Food systems issues relevant to dietetics practice can be found across the food supply chain. These problems impact the ability to produce food, food choice, and access to safe and nutritious foods. Examples in production include heavy-metal contamination of produce (Okoronkwo, Igwe, and Onwuchekwa 2005), policies like the Farm Bill that encourage the production of certain crops (Congressional Research Service 2019), and on-farm practices that degrade the soil and contribute to the emission of greenhouse gasses (Manale et al. 2018; Neff, Merrigan, and Wallinga 2015). Examples in processing include ultra-processed convenience and fast food (Juul et al. 2018), food additives and preservation (Laudisi, Stolfi, and Monteleone 2019), and food fortification and functional foods (Gul, Singh, and Jabeen 2016; Osendarp et al. 2018). Finally, examples in distribution, retail, and consumption include healthy-food availability and affordability (Pitt et al. 2017), food labeling (Shangguan et al. 2019), food advertising (Harris and Kalnova 2018), and food waste (Conrad et al. 2018). Although this is not an exhaustive list of the issues across the food system that are important for dietitians to understand, it illustrates the breadth of issues over which dietitians should have a working level of knowledge and expertise.

In the late 1980s and 1990s, there was recognition of the potential role of dietitians in learning about and participating in food systems because of the ability of dietitians to influence decisions around institutional food purchasing and to provide nutrition education to patients and clients (Clancy 1999; Gussow, Dye, and Clancy 1986; McNutt 1990). Dietary advice provided by dietitians assumes that adequate land and environmental quality exist for food production, a strong economy, a stable government, and community food security (Klitzke 1997). But advice means little without the assurance of a safe, healthy, and secure food supply. Recommendations made by dietitians emphasized the importance of knowledge of food and farm programs, reading concepts outside of nutrition science, such as agricultural and environmental science and economics, and understanding the relationship between food choice and the environment beyond food preferences (Klitzke 1997). A call for agricultural and ecological concepts within dietetics education was emphasized to avoid teaching students that "the only important part of the food system to dietetics professionals is the food choices available in the grocery store" (Klitzke 1997, 196).

The concept of "civic dietetics" came out of this early reimagining of the profession and was put forth as a way to apply Thomas Lyson's work on "civic agriculture" to the growing interest among practitioners in connecting nutrition recommendations and food choice with food systems (Wilkins 2009). Civic dietetics links traditional dietetic practice with public policy, economic development, and food system evaluation to address nutrition issues (Wilkins 2009). It assumes that "the environmental, social and economic sustainability of the system from which food is derived . . . are as relevant to food choices and dietary recommendations as nutritional quality" (Wilkins 2009, 59). It asserts that the externalities related to food choice and the political and economic forces that impact the food system are as applicable to dietetics practice as the nutritional value of foods and the relationship between dietary decisions and health. Actions associated with this concept include dietitians' ability to make recommendations for healthy diets that incorporate information on production method and environmental impacts, linking food and nutrient needs of communities with food systems by engaging varying stakeholders, and expanding evaluations of the healthfulness of food to include sustainability criteria (Wilkins 2009).

The academy has also recognized the need for dietitians to understand how food is produced and distributed. The academy (formerly the American Dietetic Association [ADA]) appointed a Sustainable Food Systems Task Force in 2005 and tasked it with the development of a primer "to increase member awareness of sustainable food systems practices and emerging roles for food and nutrition professionals in this area of practice" (ADA FST 2007, 1). The primer contained a sustainable food systems model, which highlighted the natural and human resource inputs necessary for a food system and the additional factors (i.e., values, economic, policy, research, and education) that influence food system functioning. It showed that the task force deemed sustainable food systems to be "ecologically sound, socially acceptable, and economically viable" (ADA FST 2007, 16).

In 2014, the academy hosted a conference to highlight the need for consensus around the RDN's role in global agriculture, health, and nutrition (Vogliano, Steiber, and Brown 2015). The conference attendees developed action areas for the profession, which included increasing educational opportunities for professionals around sustainability. RDN contributions to this issue were identified and included "promot[ing] sustainable farming techniques, advocat[ing] for safe and nutritious food processing, collaborat[ing] with retailers to encourage healthy options, educat[ing] consumers on evidence-based nutrition information" and included a focus on reducing food waste and increasing education around food preservation and storage (Vogliano, Steiber, and Brown 2015, 1711).

More recently, the academy emphasized food systems and sustainability in its strategic plan, position statements and practice papers, and policy priorities. In 2017, the academy's revised strategic plan included a new mission, vision, and set of principles that expanded the influence and reach of the academy and the nutrition and dietetics profession (AND n.d.[a]). Included in its food and nutrition safety and security focus is increasing access to safe and nutritious food and water, encouraging "sustainable nutrition" and healthy food systems, and leveraging creative strategies in the reduction of food waste (AND n.d.[b]). This focus is restated in its 2021 strategic plan (AND 2021c). The year 2017 also marked the academy's first revision of the Standards of Professional Performance for RDNs in Sustainable, Resilient, and Healthy Food and Water Systems, which were subsequently updated in 2020 (Spiker, Reinhardt, and Bruening 2020; Tagtow et al. 2017).

The academy's current position on sustainability states that food production, consumption, and waste impact the sustainability of the global food supply and that sustainable food systems are necessary to feed a growing population and to mitigate the effects of climate change (AND n.d.[d]). A series of position papers published by the academy beginning in 1992 highlight the importance of dietitians' understanding food system–related issues such as environmental and resource conservation and waste and the importance of their taking action in these areas (Harmon and Gerald 2007). The most recent practice paper recommends that nutrition professionals promote sustainable practices, in both their professional and personal lives, by acquiring knowledge of external costs and natural resources, implementing practices, and shaping policy (Robinson-O'Brien and Gerald 2013). A framework for action was also published, which delineated five "entry points" for nutrition professionals to interface with food system sustainability, as follows: (1) creating and implementing dietary guidance; (2) improving food, nutrition, and water security; (3) aligning nutrition and food production; (4) improving food environments and supply chains; and (5) reducing food, water, and resource waste (Spiker et al. 2020).

The academy's position on healthy food systems is supported by its policy priorities. The academy's Legislative and Public Policy Committee advocates for legislative and regulatory issues that align with the organization's strategic plan. The committee has prioritized initiatives related to food system sustainability since 2010, focusing on the Dietary Guidelines for Americans (DGAs) and the Farm Bill, among others (Blankenship and Brown 2021). The academy called for a sustainability focus in the 2020 DGAs so that adequate resources and environments exist to support availability and affordability of foods consistent with recommended dietary patterns (AND 2018). This recommendation was echoed in the academy's statement on the 2020–25 DGAs, which noted gaps in the most recently updated guidance that included recognizing the relationship between sustainability and nutrition and emphasizing the importance of food system sustainability in the DGA creation (AND 2021a). This focus and recognition has been supported by large nutrition organizations such as the Society for Nutrition Education and Behavior (Rose, Heller, and Roberto 2019). The academy's priorities for the Farm Bill, which is the largest piece of legislation that authorizes food and agriculture policy in the United States (Au et al. 2018), include promoting healthy food systems. In addition to prioritizing support for the federal food and nutrition programs in the Farm Bill, the academy recommended supporting a food supply chain that can produce healthy, safe food while reducing waste (AND n.d.[c]; Blankenship and Brown 2021). This included support for regional food systems and food access initiatives that expand the availability of regionally grown food and promote economic development (AND n.d.[c]; Blankenship and Brown 2021). It also supported policies that conserve the environment and natural resources and ensure that the next generation of farmers have access to land and skills necessary for food production (AND n.d.[c]; Blankenship and Brown 2021). Some of the specific programs supported by the academy include the Local Food Promotion Program, the Farmers Market Promotion Program, the Senior and WIC Farmers' Market Nutrition Programs, the Healthy Food Financing Initiative, and the Community Food Projects and Value Added Producer grants (AND n.d.[c]).

Food Systems in Dietetics Education

In addition to the academy, dietitians, dietetics educators, and employers recognize the importance of food systems topics, such as sustainability, in dietetics training and practice (Balch 1996; Harmon et al. 2011; Kicklighter et al. 2017; Webber and Sarjanhan 2011). Despite the increasing awareness of sustainability and dietitians' incorporation of sustainability into practice over time, less than half of dietitians report incorporating these issues into practice (Heidelberger et al. 2017). Limitations include lack of budget, limited employer support, and lack of knowledge around issues of sustainability (Hawkins, Balsam, and Graves 2015; Heidelberger et al. 2017).

The academy created the Sustainable, Resilient, and Healthy Food and Water Systems Curriculum for Dietetic Interns (SFS) in response to growing career opportunities and interest among students in sustainable food systems and the lack of time and resources cited by dietetic program directors to provide the necessary training (Hege et al. 2021). The curriculum was created for internship programs, which include one thousand supervised practice hours and coursework that are completed following undergraduate coursework in dietetics. The curriculum was piloted, revised, and released to the public in 2018 (AND 2021b; Hege et al. 2021; Knoblock-Hahn and Medrow 2020). It consists of thirteen activities that address the seven sectors of the food system as defined by the academy, including production, processing, distribution, preparation, retail, consumption, and waste management, that can be integrated into internships as rotation or program concentrations or stand-alone activities. An evaluation found that the curriculum has predominantly been used as stand-alone activities in internships with reported increased learning around its competencies. However, barriers—like time—exist in implementing the curriculum in internships and information is lacking about the use of the SFS in undergraduate dietetics programs (Hege et al. 2021).

The Accreditation Council for Education in Nutrition and Dietetics (ACEND) sets and enforces the standards for accredited university dietetics programs at the undergraduate, internship, and graduate levels and addresses the body of knowledge that university programs require students to have. In 1997, the required body of knowledge was updated to include food-related environmental issues (ACEND 2023; Gilmore, Maillet, and Mitchell 1997). Current required components in the curricula of undergraduate didactic programs in dietetics include fundamentals of public policy (including the legislative and regulatory basis of nutrition and dietetics practice), food systems, and environmental sustainability (AND n.d.[a]).

Although dietitians and nutrition professionals are engaged, to varying degrees, in ensuring a safe and healthy food supply, education to facilitate sustainable food systems and practices is not well established (Wegener and Petitclerc 2018). Despite support from the academy and current requirements of undergraduate dietetics program curricula, several challenges face the incorporation of food system-related content in dietetics programs. Faculty report feeling unprepared to teach food system topics and rank topics related to food, food choice, and food safety as more important than those related to agriculture, natural resources, and social issues (Harmon et al. 2011). These latter topics are seen as outside the purview of dietetics by many educators. Other challenges include lack of guidance on curricula, assignments/projects and research, and reading lists (Harmon et al. 2011).

Strategies for including food systems issues into undergraduate education include providing lectures, webinars, field trips, "green" dining experiences, guest speakers, fieldwork, and service learning opportunities (Wegener, Fong, and Rocha 2018). Activities included in the academy's SFS curriculum have also been suggested for inclusion in undergraduate courses (Hege et al. 2021). These strategies can be incorporated into current courses in the dietetics curriculum, most notably community nutrition, life cycle nutrition, and food service management (Harmon et al. 2011). Many examples of broader education and specific activities for students exist. Some of these include the following:

Broad education (Wilkins et al. 2010)
- Educate students about the larger ecological, economic, and political contexts of nutritional health
- Educate students about regional, sustainable food systems
- Train students in policy and advocacy related to food systems
- Educate students on ways they can engage with food systems policy and programs as dietitians

Specific activities (Harmon et al. 2011)

Community nutrition

- Visit community and school gardens
- Participate in community supported agriculture
- Examine food security in their community and advocate for policy action
- Build an understanding of sustainability and its relationship to health
- Examine how land use and planning decisions impact food availability within a community

Food service management

- Food preparation using regional and seasonal ingredients
- Meal production project that includes environmental impact and conservation considerations
- Engage in food rescue/gleaning
- Partner with local producers/community gardens to increase utilization of local foods, learn about growing practices and composting

Alternatively, new courses can be developed at universities to broaden students' knowledge of the food system and to meet the policy and sustainability competencies required of dietetics students. Several universities are already adopting new courses in their dietetics curricula that address food systems, policy, and/or society. Some of these programs include those at Auburn University, Colorado State University, the University of Alabama, UC Berkeley, Florida State University, the University of Georgia, Iowa State University, Cornell University, and New Mexico State University. As a food studies scholar, I taught a food systems course at New York University and have created a food systems and policy in dietetics course for undergraduate dietetics students at New Mexico State University.

This course draws on my research and the resources I gained during my time in the food studies program at New York University. It incorporates videos and webinars on food systems and sustainability from the academy, various universities, and organizations working on sustainability that have traditionally been seen as outside the scope of dietetics education. Texts and articles written by journalists and food advocates in addition to scholarly works from the fields of agricultural economics, environmental and agricultural sciences, public policy, public health, and nutrition are leveraged to expose students to the policy environment that shapes the US food system as well as the myriad social and economic consequences of food production and consumption. In the course, students write assessments of introduced legislation and leave-behinds on nutrition-related topics, engage in advocacy efforts around regional food systems, food security, and sustainability, and are encouraged to think critically about the relationships between food systems, policy, and dietetics practice. Weekly topics from food production to consumption engage students in discussions about current food system controversies and highlight externalities of the food system not addressed in other courses. These include impacts on workers and animal welfare throughout the food supply chain, farm inputs on human and animal health, and food processing on health. Discussions also include the impact of the food system on food availability, affordability, and waste and the information available that assists (or confuses) decisions around healthy dietary choice.

As interest in food systems grows among health professionals, educators, and the public, dietitians are poised to join the conversation. The food system and its associated "wicked problems" that impact environmental and population health is an area with growing interdisciplinary interest and collaboration. The topic provides an opportunity to enhance the critical thinking skills of future practitioners, which is valuable in all practice settings, and undergraduate programs may have the flexibility to incorporate material into existing courses or develop new courses that address multiple competencies. Food studies programs that attract scholars who examine critical questions related to food culture and systems can aid in expanding the knowledge of dietetics students beyond the traditional scope with interdisciplinary resources, activities, and readings that educators can use in the classroom. However, buy-in from dietetics educators on the importance of food systems and sustainability is imperative to evolving programs and expanding student knowledge and skills.

REFERENCES

Academy of Nutrition and Dietetics (AND). n.d.(a). "2017 Standards and Templates." Accessed June 15, 2021. https://www.eatrightpro.org.
———. n.d.(b). "The Academy's Strategic Plan." Accessed June 16, 2021. https://www.eatrightpro.org.

———. n.d.(c). "Farm Bill." Accessed June 16, 2021. https://www.eatrightpro.org.

———. n.d.(d). "Sustainable Food Systems." Accessed June 17, 2021. https://www.eatright pro.org.

———. 2018. "Academy comments to USDA and HHS re DGA Topics and Questions." Accessed June 23, 2021. https://www.eatrightpro.org.

———. 2021a. Accessed June 21, 2021. "Academy Commends Evidence-Based 2020–2025 Dietary Guidelines for Americans, Notes Opportunities for Future Updates." https://www.eatrightpro.org.

———. 2021b. Accessed June 21, 2021. "Sustainable, Resilient, and Healthy Food and Water Systems (SFS): A Curriculum for Dietetics Programs." https://eatrightfoundation.org.

———. 2021c. Accessed June 23, 2021. "Academy of Nutrition and Dietetics Strategic Plan." https://www.eatrightpro.org.

Accreditation Council for Education in Nutrition and Dietetics (ACEND). 2023. Policy and Procedure Manual. Chicago: Academy of Nutrition and Dietetics.

Almerico, Gina M. 2014. "Food and Identity: Food Studies, Cultural, and Personal Identity." Journal of International Business and Cultural Studies 8: 1.

American Dietetic Association Sustainable Food System Task Force (ADA FST). 2007. Healthy Land, Healthy People: Building a Better Understanding of Sustainable Food Systems for Food and Nutrition Professionals. A Primer on Sustainable Food Systems and Emerging Roles for Food and Nutrition Professionals. Chicago: American Dietetic Association.

Au, Lauren E., Karen Ehrens, Nicole Burda, and Erin Zumbrun. 2018. "The Academy of Nutrition and Dietetics' Priorities in the 2018 Farm Bill." Journal of the Academy of Nutrition and Dietetics 118, no. 4 (April): 767–70. https://doi.org/10.1016/j.jand.2018.01.021.

Balch, George I. 1996. "Employers' Perceptions of the Roles of Dietetics Practitioners: Challenges to Survive and Opportunities to Thrive." Journal of the American Dietetic Association 96, no. 12 (December): 1301–5. https://doi.org/10.1016/S0002-8223(96)00341-0.

Blankenship, Jeanne, and Robyn Smith Brown. 2020. "Food System Sustainability: An Academy Advocacy Priority." Journal of the Academy of Nutrition and Dietetics 120, no. 6 (June): 1054–56. https://doi.org/10.1016/j.jand.2020.02.019.

Clancy, Kate. 1999. "Reclaiming the Social and Environmental Roots of Nutrition Education." Journal of Nutrition Education 31, no. 4 (July): 190–93. https://doi.org/10.1016/S0022-3182(99)70440-1.

Congressional Research Service. 2019. 2018 Farm Bill (P.L. 115–334) Primer Series: A Guide to Omnibus Farm and Food Legislation. CRS Report R45984. Accessed June 13, 2021. https://crsreports.congres.gov.

Conrad, Zach, Meredith T. Niles, Deborah A. Neher, Eric D. Roy, Nicole E. Tichenor, and Lisa Jahns. 2018. "Relationship between Food Waste, Diet Quality, and Environmental Sustainability." PLOS ONE 13 (4): e0195405. https://doi.org/10.1371/journal.pone.0195405

Gandy, Joan, ed. 2019. Manual of Dietetic Practice. Hoboken, NJ: Wiley-Blackwell.

Gilmore, Carol J., Julie O'Sullivan Maillet, and Beverly E. Mitchell. "Determining Educational Preparation Based on Job Competencies of Entry-Level Dietetics Practitioners." *Journal of the Academy of Nutrition and Dietetics* 97, no. 3 (1997): 306.

Gul, Khalid, A. K. Singh, and Rifat Jabeen. 2016. "Nutraceuticals and Functional Foods: The Foods for the Future World." *Critical Reviews in Food Science and Nutrition* 56 (16): 2617–27. https://doi.org/10.1080/10408398.2014.903384.

Gussow, Joan Dye, and Katherine L. Clancy. 1986. "Dietary Guidelines for Sustainability." *Journal of Nutrition Education* 18, no. 1 (February): 1–5. https://doi.org/10.1016/S0022-3182(86)80255-2.

Hamm, Michael W. "Principles for Framing a Healthy Food System." 2009. *Journal of Hunger & Environmental Nutrition* 4 (3–4): 241–50. https://doi.org/10.1080/19320240903321219.

Harmon, Alison H., and Bonnie L. Gerald. 2007. "Position of the American Dietetic Association: Food and Nutrition Professionals can Implement Practices to Conserve Natural Resources and Support Ecological Sustainability." *Journal of the American Dietetic Association* 107, no. 6 (June): 1033–43. https://doi.org/10.1016/j.jada.2007.04.018.

Harmon, Alison, Julia L. Lapp, Dorothy Blair, and Annie Hauck-Lawson. 2011. "Teaching Food System Sustainability in Dietetic Programs: Need, Conceptualization, and Practical Approaches." *Journal of Hunger & Environmental Nutrition* 6 (1): 114–24. https://doi.org/10.1080/19320248.2011.554272.

Harris, Jennifer L., and Svetlana S. Kalnova. 2018. "Food and Beverage TV Advertising to Young Children: Measuring Exposure and Potential Impact." *Appetite* 123, no. 1 (April): 49–55. https://doi.org/10.1016/j.appet.2017.11.110.

Hawkins, Irana W., Alan L. Balsam, and Daren Graves. 2015. "A Qualitative Study of How Registered Dietitians Made the Connection Between Diet, Climate Change, and Environmental Degradation." *Journal of Hunger & Environmental Nutrition* 10 (1): 47–59. https://doi.org/10.1080/19320248.2015.1004213.

Hege, Amanda, Janice Giddens, Erin Bergquist, Diane Stadler, Christina Gayer Campbell, Joanna Cummings, Anne Goetze et al. 2021. "Integration of a Sustainable Food Systems Curriculum in Nutrition and Dietetics Education: Assessment From the First Year of Implementation." *Journal of the Academy of Nutrition and Dietetics* S2212–2672, no. 21 (December): 00074–5. https://doi.org/10.1016/j.jand.2021.02.001.

Heidelberger, Lindsay, Chery Smith, Ramona Robinson-O'Brien, Carrie Earthman, and Kim Robien. 2017. "Registered Dietitian Nutritionists' Perspectives on Integrating Food and Water System Issues into Professional Practice." *Journal of the Academy of Nutrition and Dietetics* 117, no. 2 (February): 271–77. https://doi.org/10.1016/j.jand.2016.06.380.

Juul, Filippa, Euridice Martinez-Steele, Niyati Parekh, Carlos A. Monteiro, and Virginia W. Chang. 2018. "Ultra-Processed Food Consumption and Excess Weight Among US Adults." *British Journal of Nutrition* 120 (1): 90–100. https://doi.org/10.1017/S0007114518001046.

Kicklighter, Jana R., Becky Dorner, Anne Marie Hunter, Marcy Kyle, Melissa Pflugh Prescott, Susan Roberts, Bonnie Spear, Rosa K Hand, and Cecily Byrne. 2017. "Visioning Report 2017: A Preferred Path Forward for the Nutrition and Dietetics Profession." *Journal of the Academy of Nutrition and Dietetics* 117, no. 1 (January): 110–27. https://doi.org/10.1016/j.jand.2016.09.027.

Klitzke, Carol. 1997. "Dietitians: Experts about Food Systems?" *Journal of the American Dietetic Association* 97, no. 10 (October): S195–96. https://doi.org/10.1016/s0002-8223(97)00763-3.

Knoblock-Hahn, Amy, and Lisa Medrow. 2020. "Development and Implementation of a Sustainable, Resilient, and Healthy Food and Water Systems Curriculum for Dietetic Interns." *Journal of the Academy of Nutrition and Dietetics* 120, no. 1 (January): 130–33. https://doi.org/10.1016/j.jand.2019.04.016.

Kreuter, Marshall W., Christopher De Rosa, Elizabeth H. Howze, and Grant T. Baldwin. 2004. "Understanding Wicked Problems: A Key to Advancing Environmental Health Promotion." *Health Education & Behavior* 31, no. 4 (August): 441–54. https://doi.org/10.1177/1090198104265597.

Laudisi, Federica, Carmine Stolfi, and Giovanni Monteleone. 2019. "Impact of Food Additives on Gut Homeostasis." *Nutrients* 11, no. 10 (October): 2334. https://doi.org/10.3390/nu11102334.

Manale, Andrew, Andrew Sharpley, Catherine DeLong, David Speidel, Clark Gantzer, John Peterson, Rex Martin, Clare Lindahl, and Naveen Adusumilli. 2018. "Principles and Policies for Soil and Water Conservation." *Journal of Soil and Water Conservation* 73, no. 4 (July): 96A–99A. https://doi.org/10.2489/jswc.73.4.96A.

McNutt, Kristen. 1990. "Integrating Nutrition and Environmental Objectives." *Nutrition Today* 25, no. 6 (November): 40–41.

Miller, Jeffrey P., and Jonathan Deutsch. 2009. *Food Studies: An Introduction to Research Methods.* New York: Berg.

Neff, Roni A., Kathleen Merrigan, and David Wallinga. 2015. "A Food Systems Approach to Healthy Food and Agriculture Policy." *Health Affairs (Millwood)* 34, no. 11 (November): 1908–15. https://doi.org/10.1377/hlthaff.2015.0926.

Nestle, Marion, and W. Alex McIntosh. 2010. "Writing the Food Studies Movement." *Food, Culture & Society* 13 (2): 159–79. https://doi.org/10.2752/175174410X12633934462999.

Okoronkwo, N. E., J. C. Igwe, and E. C. Onwuchekwa. 2005. "Risk and Health Implications of Polluted Soils for Crop Production." *African Journal of Biotechnology* 4 (13): 1521–24. https://www.ajol.info/index.php/ajb/issue/view/8594.

Osendarp, Saskia JM, Homero Martinez, Greg S. Garrett, Lynnette M. Neufeld, Luz Maria De-Regil, Marieke Vossenaar, and Ian Darnton-Hill. 2018. "Large-Scale Food Fortification and Biofortification in Low-and Middle-Income Countries: A Review of Programs, Trends, Challenges, and Evidence Gaps." *Food and Nutrition Bulletin* 39, no. 2 (May): 315–31. https://doi.org/10.1177/0379572118774229.

Pitt, Erin, Danielle Gallegos, Tracy Comans, Cate Cameron, and Lukar Thornton. 2017. "Exploring the Influence of Local Food Environments on Food Behaviours:

A Systematic Review of Qualitative Literature." *Public Health Nutrition* 20, no. 13 (June): 2393–2405. https://doi.org/10.1017/S1368980017001069.

Robinson-O'Brien, Ramona, and Bonnie L Gerald. 2013. "Practice Paper of the Academy of Nutrition and Dietetics Abstract: Promoting Ecological Sustainability Within the Food System." *Journal of the Academy of Nutrition and Dietetics* 113, no. 3 (March): 464. https://doi.org/10.1016/j.jand.2013.01.016.

Rose, Donald, Martin C. Heller, and Christina A. Roberto. 2019. "Position of the Society for Nutrition Education and Behavior: The Importance of Including Environmental Sustainability in Dietary Guidance." *Journal of Nutrition Education and Behavior* 51 no. 1: 3–15. https://doi.org/10.1016/j.jneb.2018.07.006

Shangguan, Siyi, Ashkan Afshin, Masha Shulkin, Wenjie Ma, Daniel Marsden, Jessica Smith, Michael Saheb-Kashaf et al. 2019. "A Meta-Analysis of Food Labeling Effects on Consumer Diet Behaviors and Industry Practices." *American Journal of Preventive Medicine* 56, no. 2 (January): 300–14. https://doi.org/10.1016/j.amepre.2018.09.024.

Spiker, Marie L, Amy Knoblock-Hahn, Katie Brown, James Giddens, Amanda S Hege, Kevin Sauer, Diane M Enos, and Alison Steiber. 2020. "Cultivating Sustainable, Resilient, and Healthy Food and Water Systems: A Nutrition-Focused Framework for Action." *Journal of the Academy of Nutrition and Dietetics* 120, no. 6 June): 1057–67. https://doi.org/10.1016/j.jand.2020.02.018.

Spiker, Marie, Sarah Reinhardt, and Meg Bruening. 2020. "Academy of Nutrition and Dietetics: Revised 2020 Standards of Professional Performance for Registered Dietitian Nutritionists (Competent, Proficient, and Expert) in Sustainable, Resilient, and Healthy Food and Water Systems." *Journal of the Academy of Nutrition and Dietetics* 120, no. 9 (September): 1568–85. https://doi.org/10.1016/j.jand.2020.05.010.

Tagtow Angie, Kim Robien, Erin Bergquist, Meg Bruening, Lisa Dierks, Barbara E Hartman, Ramona Robinson-O'Brien, Tamara Steinitz, Bettina Tahsin, Teri Underwood, and Jennifer Wilkins. 2014. "Academy of Nutrition and Dietetics: Standards of Professional Performance for Registered Dietitian Nutritionists (Competent, Proficient, and Expert) in Sustainable, Resilient, and Healthy Food and Water Systems." *Journal of the Academy of Nutrition and Dietetics* 114, no. 3 (March): 475–88. https://doi.org/10.1016/j.jand.2013.11.011.

Vogliano, Chris, Alison Steiber, and Katie Brown. 2015. "Linking Agriculture, Nutrition, and Health: The Role of the Registered Dietitian Nutritionist." *Journal of the Academy of Nutrition and Dietetics* 115, no. 10 (October): 1710–14. https://doi.org/10.1016/j.jand.2015.06.009.

Webber, Caroline B., and Andy Sarjahani. 2011. "Fitting Sustainable Food Systems into Dietetic Internships—A Growing Trend." *Journal of Hunger & Environmental Nutrition* 6 (4): 477–89. https://doi.org/10.1080/19320248.2011.627304.

Wegener, Jessica. 2018. "Equipping Future Generations of Registered Dietitian Nutritionists and Public Health Nutritionists: A Commentary on Education and Training Needs to Promote Sustainable Food Systems and Practices in the 21st Century."

Journal of the Academy of Nutrition and Dietetics 118, no. 3 (March): 393–98. https://doi.org/10.1016/j.jand.2017.10.024.

Wegener, Jessica, Debbie Fong, and Cecilia Rocha. 2018. "Education, Practical Training and Professional Development for Public Health Practitioners: A Scoping Review of the Literature and Insights for Sustainable Food System Capacity-Building." *Public Health Nutrition* 21, no. 9 (February): 1771–80. https://doi.org/10.1017/S1368980017004207.

Wegener, Jessica, and Marilyne Petitclerc. 2018. "Opportunities and Challenges for Practical Training in Public Health: Insights from Practicum Coordinators in Ontario." *Canadian Journal of Dietetic Practice and Research* 79, no. 4 (December): 176–80. https://doi.org/10.3148/cjdpr-2018-014.

Wilkins, Jennifer L. 2009. "Civic Dietetics: Opportunities for Integrating Civic Agriculture Concepts into Dietetic Practice." *Agriculture and Human Values* 26 (1–2): 57–66. https://doi.org/10.1007/s10460-008-9177-2.

Wilkins, Jennifer L., Julia Lapp, Angie Tagtow, and Susan Roberts. 2010. "Beyond Eating Right: The Emergence of Civic Dietetics to Foster Health and Sustainability through Food System Change." *Journal of Hunger & Environmental Nutrition* 5 (1): 2–12. https://doi.org/10.1080/19320240903573983.

8

Culinary Arts

Practicing Food while Practicing Food Studies

JONATHAN M. DEUTSCH

Personal Stance: My Inner Evil

When I began my graduate studies at NYU in 1999, Marion Nestle was in the throes of writing *Food Politics*. While Amy Bentley was my advisor and the supervisor for my graduate assistantship, she was a new assistant professor and appropriately deferential to the department chair and *grande dame* of food studies, occasionally "lending" me to assist with *Food Politics*. Working with Marion, I discovered my inner evil. I never knew it existed. I thought I was a nice Jewish boy—it's what my mom always called me.

When I was a reluctant serial bar mitzvah attendee, I gravitated toward the kitchen of the synagogue, where desserts could be snuck before the appointed time, and where the shammash was always happy to have some boys around to help with the dishes. I became hooked on the kitchen and decided then to have a career as a chef, where I could eat with gusto (I grew up in a household where the menus could be described as dietetic at best) and not ossify at a desk job. I started dishwashing and then cooking professionally as soon as I got my working papers at fourteen and committed to attend the Culinary Institute of America, over the objections of my guidance counselor, who pleaded that I was on the "academic track" and therefore should consider a hospitality management program at one of our nation's fine land-grant universities. I cooked in a variety of settings—institutional foodservice, wholesale pasta maker, restaurant, caterer—and went on to intern at Nestlé's (the company, not the scholar) international R&D center, where I stayed on on a project basis.

Upon enrolling in the food studies PhD program at NYU, Nestle's (the scholar, not the company) work revealed that I was a member of the evil agri-industrial complex. All this time doing fat reductions, cost reductions, and new product development for familiar brands of cheese sauce, canned vegetables, and TV dinners, it never occurred to me that others could see this tedious benchtop formulation as contributing to the dysfunction of the conventional food system. My corporate take on Thai red curry was lackluster, its spice level dialed to just one click above Stroganoff (per marketing's brief); its umami flavors, from allergens like dried shrimp or fish sauce, unceremoniously removed (per guidance from risk management and regulatory compliance); and its prep, cooked to a temperature that would ensure that cryophilic bacteria would not even *dream* of hanging out in your supermarket's freezer section (thanks to food safety and engineering), providing the culinary coup de grace. But *evil?* As I read more of Marion's work and the sources she cited, I learned that I was not the nice boy I thought I was. I was complicit in causing obesity, non-communicable diseases, the decline of the family farm, cancer among farmworkers, animal cruelty, and ultimately the environmental degradation leading to the extinction of the human species. That's a lot for a young graduate student to bear (though maybe I didn't need to take things quite so personally).

At the same time, I have fondness for so many of my food industry colleagues, whose goals, it may shock food studies scholars to know, were not to end civilization, catalyze climate change, or obfuscate its production practices from the conscious consumer but rather to make safe and affordable food products (and food has never been safer or more affordable, despite its problems), avoid being laid off in the increased consolidation of the food industry, afford to send their kids to college, and retire at sixty-five to travel to enjoy the gold standard versions of pastries, pastas, salsas, and empanadas, a.k.a. "hot pockets," that they had spent their careers bastardizing.

It is at this intersection of being *in* and *of* the conventional food system from my professional work in the industry, and the critical study of the food system in food studies, that I will explore in this chapter.

Thematic Tension

It seems there are two distinct camps in the academic study of food: (1) programs teaching people to be complicit actors in the dysfunctional conventional food system as professional food scientists, chefs, veterinarians, marketers, entrepreneurs, farmers, retailers, supply chain managers, agro-economists, food safety consultants, and so on; and (2) programs teaching people to be critical of the people in (1), the work they do, and the policies, structures, and markets enabling them to do it, as public health and policy advocates, nutritionists, sustainable agriculture advocates, rural sociologists, and food studies scholars, to name a few. Students in (1) aspire to jobs producing food as farmers, ranchers, or food processors, buying that food as wholesalers, retailers, restaurateurs, or foodservice managers, or supporting the food industry providing research, consulting, marketing, financing, or other services. Students in (2) aspire to spend their efforts repairing the damage caused by the people in (1) as social workers, health workers, nutritionists, environmentalists, and educators; advocating for regulations or policy changes to make (1) work better, or piloting alternative food system interventions to model how (1) can work better, to name a few. And of course, there is a messy middle—sustainable food companies, artisanal food producers, food hubs, urban farms, ethical retailers, and similar organizations that straddle the practical food provisioning and the critical lens in order to feed well while doing good.

It is in the space in between where I've been working, reconciling my pre-NYU studies and experiences learning how to excel in the extant system ("Oui, Chef!"), with my NYU studies that trained me to consider the true cost of that system to planet and people, remembering all of their identities and intersectionalities ("Why, Chef?") (Deutsch 2016).

Shortly before I graduated from NYU, I took my first full-time teaching job, founding and teaching in the culinary arts program at Kingsborough Community College of the City University of New York. Marion was unenthusiastic ("A community college?!"). But we had a baby on the way (who is now a college student herself), so it was time to move from graduate student assistant to academic employee, and I was drawn to the public mission, the students, colleagues, and beachfront campus near Coney Island. There I combined both my schools of study. By day, I taught students to be food professionals: food safety, guest services, knife skills, stocks, sauces, cooking methods, and so on, with only the faintest whiff, where the curriculum and schedule allowed, for critique of the culinary profession and its practices, with a bit more emphasis on impending food system problems and challenges. By night, I was a teaching assistant at NYU and wrote a dissertation about food and masculinities, with all its requisite problematizing and intersecting, although with just barely enough problematizing and intersecting to appease Amy Bentley and Krishnendu Ray, both on my committee.

I continued that bifurcated life through twelve years at Kingsborough, teaching cooking and consulting to the food industry on food product development by day, while churning out books and articles on improving food studies and culinary education and food and culture that were needed for academic deliverance by night.

Epiphany: Thematic Integration

While I dabbled with combining these worlds—introducing canonical food studies concepts like Hauck-Lawson's food voice (2006) in my table service classes or having students design a "better" school lunch menu in a course on food service management—teaching food to developing future food professionals and thinking critically about food remained parallel tracks for me, two important and rarely entangling legs of the tenure stool, teaching and research.

In 2013, I took an opportunity to teach food and hospitality at my undergraduate alma mater, Drexel University. There, a couple of factors conspired to challenge me to think differently about my bifurcated life. The first consideration was simply practical: I was too busy recovering from the whiplash of moving from a community college to a Carnegie R1 research university to keep up the industry consulting side of my identity. The pace of Drexel, which operates year-round on ten-week quarters, is intense, leaving little time for gigging. The second factor was the students. Even though the curricula at Drexel and Kingsborough were similar from the practicalities of delivering content—calculating food cost, dicing an onion, solving guest problems, reading a restaurant P&L, for example—the students were frequently doing something that my Kingsborough students hadn't done: questioning. It would be an inaccurate generalization to say that my Drexel students were smarter than my Kingsborough students and, in fact, some were my students at both institutions. But the type of intelligence each group has is different. At Kingsborough, students were hungry for learning and opportunity. Students overwhelmingly understood that I had some things (knowledge, experience, and cultural capital) that they needed access and replicate in order to better their own professional career paths. Their job was to get it. At Drexel, especially at the upper-division and graduate level, students had (or thought they had) plenty of their own knowledge and experience. As for cultural capital, it is hard to flex to a student whose apartment is a suite at the Ritz Carlton or who has eaten at great restaurants in every city with an NBA franchise since her boyfriend is "on the team." They didn't need—or thought they didn't need—to unlock the store of knowledge, experience, and cultural capital in my head. The main difference I perceived with the Drexel students was their commitment to questioning—*Why* are we doing it this way? *Why* are things so bad in various situations in our community and food system? *How* can I help? What we might call a critical food studies lens was not shaped by an altruistic commitment to improving the food system; rather, it referenced the students' perception that they were valued and empowered members of an engaged citizenry where they had the right to question and improve their own situation and the situation of as others. Rather than seeing themselves as vessels to be filled with information, my Drexel students asserted themselves as aspiring peers with a commitment to one day being my colleague—if not my boss—in the culinary community,.

In my early teaching at Drexel, I similarly divided the practical aspects of culinary arts (culinary skills classes) from food studies and food systems–oriented classes, as was my training. Bananas changed all that. The epiphany for me of how I needed to do things differently at Drexel—and also how to integrate the two disparate sides of my own professional life, cooking and food studies—came on a tour of a food-waste prevention and recovery initiative, led by the EPA. It is a story I've told numerous times and refer to as "the banana story."

Shortly after starting at Drexel, the US Environmental Protection Agency (EPA) reached out with an opportunity. The neighborhood surrounding the university is one of great disparity. There are anchor institutions like universities, hospitals, supermarkets, and transit hubs, side by side with one of the poorest residential neighborhoods in the country. The EPA found it unconscionable that there would be food insecurity side-by-side with abundance. Working with urban planning students [focused on food systems], the EPA developed a program where community-based organizations could pick up discards of safe, edible foods (from anchor institutions) to take them back to their sites. Often, the most perishable foods were the most nutritious and most needed for health promotion—foods like bananas, leafy greens, berries, and milk. Our students shadowed the donation process and followed these still-edible, safe, and wholesome foods from the supermarket donation system to the site, a local shelter for women and children.

At one lunch, rice and chicken came from the city's Office of Homeless Services, a salad appeared with the lettuce, tomatoes, and carrots donated from the supermarket, bottled ranch dressing was purchased at a club store, and there was a donated cake for dessert. At the end of the buffet was a large stainless steel bowl of (donated) bananas, about one per person.

As we watched the women and their children move through the buffet, we saw plenty of smiles and heard appreciative comments. They piled plates with rice, chicken, salad, and generous hunks of cake. But when they got to the bananas, there were only a few takers. Four (out of fifty), to be exact.

At the end of the meal, the chef packed up leftovers to be used in case someone missed a meal. About a dozen bananas stayed out for snacking with the cake. The remainder went to the dumpster. Tomorrow there would be a new case of bananas.

While the urban planning/food systems students were counting pounds of food rescued from the waste stream and declaring victory that fresh fruits and vegetables were being redirected to a vulnerable population that needed it most, our culinary students saw something very different: waste moving around the food system. They also saw flavor and nutrition going to waste. Like a rock on a cliff full of potential energy, the fruit on the precipice of the dumpster is potentially delicious food. But with all good intentions, the shelter was subsidizing the waste management costs of the supermarket by taking their surplus and moving it to their own dumpster, without the benefit of a composting program and the financial resources to accommodate.

Seeing this, our students developed a simple and elegant solution: a banana "ice cream," made with as few as one ingredient (banana) and potentially more. The process was simple—peel and freeze the bananas on sheet trays. Using a mixer, food processor, or even a hand-held potato masher, puree the frozen bananas until an ice cream-like texture is achieved. This is not a novel recipe—banana "whip" recipes abound. But by applying it to this particular setting, our students could raise the consumption of bananas from a few a day overall to the full case and even more.

This food intervention had a few positive outcomes: increased fruit consumption in a vulnerable population and a reduction in food waste, most obviously. But there is one outcome that is less tangible: a social and emotional shift in the food voice (Hauck-Lawson 2006) from the bowl of bananas saying, "Here are some healthy overripe leftovers from the supermarket if anyone would like one," to a volunteer scooping a smooth frozen treat saying, "Would anyone like some ice cream?" A cultural shift achieved through simple cooking.

Seeing students apply the practical menu development-oriented culinary skills they learn in their practical classes to a food-systems problem was an epiphany for me. It led to a research agenda focused on reforming culinary education to not simply produce ethical technicians of the future but also to be sure that chefs and food scientists are at the table in addressing food system problems (Deutsch 2016).

Drexel Food Lab

Based on these formative experiences and others, a then undergraduate student, Alexandra Zeitz, and I formed the Drexel Food Lab in the spring of 2014. The lab is a translational food-product-development and culinary-innovation lab focused on engaging culinary students and faculty in solving real-world problems in the areas of sustainability, health promotion, and access. Our principles our simple:

- Do good. All our projects have a social mission, one food studies scholars would recognize as aligned with their interests.
- Feed well. Taste is key. We are not pushing for policy changes or regulations. While not opposed to that, there are much better advocates than us for a better food system. We want to produce food that is eaten on its own merits.

- Keep going. All our projects need to achieve financial sustainability without subsidies or incentives for people to eat them. The market needs to demand them in some way.

Since our founding, the lab has worked on projects including upcycled foods (from food that would otherwise be wasted), food alternatives to pharmaceuticals, and improving institutional food options, among many others. We have done this work for companies ranging from startups to some of the same allegedly "evil" multinational food corporations I learned to decry in my graduate studies, as well as non-profits and government agencies including the Centers for Disease Control and municipal health departments, both in the United States and abroad.

Concluding Plea

As we enter the third decade of maturity for the NYU food studies program—what would be the prime of adulthood were our program a person—I think it is important to remember our roots and, like the Drexel Food Lab does, consistently integrate practical culinary arts and food science skills with food systems improvements. If decade 1 was establishing food culture and food systems as a legitimate academic field worthy of study in its own right, and decade 2 was showing that food studies and food studies perspectives can produce top-quality work across the humanities and social sciences, as my fellow contributors to this volume have shown, decade 3 should be the decade of "so what?" So we should eat more sustainably? Don't just talk about it, do it. Show us how.

With existing coursework in nutrition and food science and strong relationships with culinary schools and chefs (including many food studies students and alumni), food studies can and should add producing good food for the marketplace to its repertoire of pilot programs, advocacy, and critical analysis. Those who "do" food can learn to engage more fully and thoughtfully with food culture and food systems issues. Those who "speak" food can do so with their hands along with their words. From my perch in the middle, I'm honored to be part of the movement.

REFERENCES

Deutsch, Jonathan. 2016. "Revolutionizing Culinary Education: Can Cooking Save the Food System," *Proceedings of the 2016 Dublin Gastronomy Symposium.* Available at https://arrow.tudublin.ie/cgi/viewcontent.cgi?article=1098&context=dgs.

Hauck-Lawson, Annie. 2006. "All in the Family: New York Food Voice Narratives." *Appetite* 47, no. 3 (November): 390. https://doi.org/10.1016/j.appet.2006.08.024.

ACKNOWLEDGMENT

An expanded version of the banana story appears as "Shaping the Material: Turning the Food Studies Lens on Itself in Pursuit of 'Better' Food," in *The Bloomsbury Handbook of Food and Material Cultures,* ed. Elizabeth Zanoni and Irina Mihalache (New York: Bloomsbury, 2023), 41–56.

Thanks to my colleagues Alexandra Zeitz, Edward Bottone, Erica Friedman, and fellow NYU food studies alums James Feustel and Babette Audant for shaping this approach.

Technology and Applied Sciences

The last section, "Technology and Applied Sciences," points to the potential of food studies to expand beyond the confines of established academia toward new areas such as design, network science, and library sciences, as well as provide the basis for technology startups and entrepreneurship.

Technology's formal definition is the application of knowledge to reach practical goals in a specifiable and reproducible way. It is the application of scientific knowledge for a specific, even useful purpose, thus the term *applied sciences* (engineering and medicine, for example, are both classified as applied sciences). A hallmark of NYU food studies is its applied nature, in the sense of *techne*, the Greek word connoting knowledge in the context of making or doing. Knowledge is created through process.

The essays here examine (humanities/social science-based) food studies as applied to technology (cooking applications, design) and manipulating large data sets (network science and library science). It features authors who are dexterous with digital technology, work with large data sets, employ quantitative methods, or wield computer science expertise. Here food studies intersects with *digital humanities*, a catch-all phrase representing the myriad ways in which digital technologies and humanities interrelate and that includes blogging, mapping, data visualization, interactive websites, gaming, exhibits, and social media.

In the penultimate chapter, "Action Research and Social Engagement," several of us share experiences in our applied engagement with civil society and the community around us. A main tenet of NYU food studies has been locating our work at the intersection of theoretical and applied knowledge. Food is such a visceral, material, ephemeral object that it lends itself to sitting in this space. We theorize and also get our hands dirty in application and lived experience, which sets us apart from traditional academic disciplines. Part academic, part applied, we sit in this space that comfortably engages both. This extends beyond objective academic scholarship and incorporates participatory action as within academic inquiry. In the final chapter, Krishnendu Ray closes the collection with his concluding observations.

9

Startups and Entrepreneurship

Recipes, Know-How, and the Assumed Progress of Man

GRACE CHOI

There is a common belief among proficient cooks that prior to execut-
ing a dish from a written recipe for the first time, one must read through
the list of ingredients and instructions at least twice, and ideally thrice.
The idea behind this is, of course, to ensure that one has all the components and materials required, as well as to take note of the sequence
of steps and procedures. Among the more skilled, I imagine there is a
mental choreography that plays out in their imagination while reading,
especially if they are cooking multiple dishes at once. Even as a culinary
student at the now-defunct French Culinary Institute in New York City,
my final examination was based on the extent to which I could reproduce and prepare a written recipe from memory with exactness. There is
a sense of tacit inevitability that surrounds written recipes; indeed, one
marker of culinary proficiency is the ability to decipher terminologies
and interpret and reference texts for the purposes of fulfilling the action-
based endeavor that is cooking.

The question I pose, both in this essay and in my own work as the
founder of an early startup called Larabee, is whether the conventional-
ized recipe format to which we are accustomed meets the demands and
capabilities of the world we live in now. M. F. K. Fisher writes in her
essay "The Anatomy of a Recipe" (1983):

> The reasons for the gradual changes in a basic recipe such as one for
> wheat bread, for instance, *are inextricably tangled with man's history
> and assumed progress.* A thing like soup, which Jacob sold to Esau for
> his birthright in the first Biblical reference to the restaurant trade, is too
> vague to trace unless one settles definitely on the *kind* of soup, in this case

a pottage of lentils, but really the method of making a good lentil soup, even as a loaf of good bread, has changed very little in the several thousand years since it was first mentioned. It is only in the way of writing the recipe itself that has evolved, to be trimmed to our *changing tempo of reading, preparing, producing.* (14, italics added)

Fisher, in her historical timeline, attributes Dr. William Kitchiner with bestowing upon the world the beginnings of a systematic framework for recipes consisting of "exact measurements for every ingredient of a dish, as well as the order of their use." Kitchiner's book, *The Cook's Oracle; and Housekeeper's Manual*, was first published in 1822 and did away with the ambiguity and "rule of thumb"-ness of the old receipt books that preceded them, which contained language like "Work ye Butter to a cream with your hands, then put in your sugar and almonds . . . it will take four hours in a quick oven to bake it" (Fisher 1983, 17). Part of the reason Kitchiner's modifications resonated was because the audience for recipes was expanding from housekeepers to housewives and laypersons and demonstrating increased literacy. As we cross the two-hundredth anniversary of *The Cook's Oracle*, is it not time to consider whether the "assumed progress" of our current age, and the spread of what is now digital literacy, should compel us to reimagine the architecture of recipes once more?

It goes without saying that written recipes and cookbooks are uniquely important forms of literature in that they, like language, serve not only a denotative purpose but also a connotative function producing and sustaining social conventions—arguments that have been articulated by Arjun Appadurai in "How to Make a National Cuisine" (1988). More specifically, recipes deliver practical information, index social stratification among communities, particularly in class, gender, and ethnicity, indicate social situations and notions of identity, and reify cultural norms, behaviors, and attitudes. Perhaps it is now worth questioning how effective following a written recipe is in practice, particularly with regards to how human beings approach novel activities and absorb knowledge. "If you think about it," historian Ken Albala said to me over the phone, "written recipes are attempts to convert actions into words that then have to be converted back into actions."

This essay dives into my consideration of recipe frameworks and delivery in light of the technologies and innovations that gain ubiquity in our everyday lives. It is not to argue that written recipes should be rendered obsolete by the technological capabilities of the day, any more than written recipes threaten to displace in-person learning. Rather, it is to explore the best use-case for technology and design to support the drive human beings have to be generative, creative, knowledgeable, social, and part of something larger than themselves. Against the backdrop of entrepreneurship and applied food studies, I revisit critical learnings from my time as a doctoral student that have directly informed the conceptualization and design of what is now my startup, Larabee.

Applied Food Studies in the Wild

Larabee is a smart-knowledge platform that uses advanced technology and pioneering design to deliver a different way of gaining know-how. It began as an idea in 2017, a few years after completing my doctorate, while I was holding a sleeping infant to my chest and whisper-shouting commands to Amazon's voice assistant, Alexa, to play music. At the time, voice assistants were just beginning to gain ubiquity in American households, video screens and advanced features had not yet been introduced, and I had quickly grown reliant on my Echo device to set timers and fill rooms with ambient noise. Cradling my daughter's head with one hand and her bottom with the other, I wondered in that moment if there was such a thing as voice-narrated recipes, which turned into a question of whether a company that produced them might hire someone like me, which morphed into an idea that perhaps I could be the one to start one such company, which eventually turned into the realization that voice-narrated recipes was an obvious but ultimately limited idea and that there were greater opportunities afoot.

For years prior, I had been niggled by a sense of aimlessness and unease that came from not knowing my place in the world, like a boat without a rudder or an ant without a colony. The perfect descriptor is the Korean word *dap-dap-hae* (답답해), a stifling, almost suffocating sense of frustration that I equate with the inability to exhale completely into oneself. There were ways to keep busy and productive—degrees, pursuits in culinary arts and food media, family—but these felt like disparate threads in a fragmented life. I was as certain of the kinds of work I was ill-equipped for or incurious about as I was ignorant of what I wanted to do. With this new and inchoate idea, however, and the opportunity to create something that did not yet exist in the world, there arose an awareness that my path leading to this point had not been as itinerant or indeliberate as I had feared. Moreover, any sort of reimagination and actualization of culinary knowledge delivery in the manner I envisioned would have been exceptionally harder, if not impossible, had it not been for the intersections of research and discovery across food studies, applied psychology, and anthropology during my time at NYU.

From subsequent conversations, interviews, observations of teaching and learning styles at my former culinary school, immersion in the voice technology space, and analysis of videotaped sessions of myself giving recipe instruction to friends, I learned two things. First, emerging technologies made it very possible to create a scalable voice- and video-assisted recipe framework for home cooks. Second, my direct competitors were Amazon and Google. In November of 2019, Tech-Crunch announced that both companies were preparing to "double down on hands-free recipes to help sell their smart displays." One of many punches to the gut during this early period of entrepreneurship, of dreams nearly extinguished and visions for a future almost trampled before taking flight, this news was mitigated by the discovery that what these tech giants were putting out into the world was (in my very biased opinion) not great.

These hands-free recipe experiences consist of voice-activated step-by-step instructions and video demonstration, designed such that home cooks no longer have to wash their hands after handling raw chicken to refer back to their cookbooks or struggle to find their place within a long sequence of text-heavy steps, among other features. The value of this kind of convenience and ease cannot be overstated and have been integral components of Larabee's interactive design from the beginning, as they address real and expressed pain points. This, however, is not enough to draw home cooks away from the resources to which they are accustomed. Interpreting text-heavy instructions, scrolling up and down blogs to find the information one needs, filtering through countless videos to piece together a knife technique—these are frustrations and

STARTUPS AND ENTREPRENEURSHIP | 129

annoyances so prevalent they have turned into memes. Yet the home cooks I have spoken to and observed still take comfort in familiarity. They feel rooted by the permanence of text and are accustomed to darting their eyes up, down, and around recipe instructions and ingredient quantities. The real opportunity here is to create a mode of recipe guidance that captures the learner's imagination, not by iterating on what already exists but by ensuring that they feel at once supported, enlivened, and delighted. The remainder of this essay weaves together the intellectual arguments and pure imaginings that originated during my time at NYU and continue to evolve to inform Larabee's interactive framework.

Recipes and Resources in the Twenty-First Century

Let us start with the assumption that human beings want to cook. There are those for whom the act of cooking is a taxing and undesirable chore to be avoided or completed as quickly as possible, as well as many self-professed lovers of the craft who have days where nothing is less enticing. But as a broad statement, we can posit that cooking is a fundamental activity that endures in the nature of our species despite any technological advancements or marketing campaigns that say otherwise. It may seem silly to begin here given this book's audience, but I do so because, before the COVID-19 pandemic validated this claim with the force of a cartoon anvil, I heard from countless would-be investors that the practice of cooking was becoming increasingly obsolete. To them, the evidence was the trajectory from frozen meals to takeout delivery services like DoorDash and UberEats. As food studies scholars are aware, the venture capitalists who pushed back against the notion that cooking was and remains foundational to the human experience are far from alone or original in their opinions. Laura Shapiro touches on this attitude in her book *Something from the Oven*, where she discusses an advertisement from a frozen food journal from the 1950s titled "Fantasy of the Future," describing cooking and kitchens as remnants of the past. "[S]cience has emancipated women right out of the kitchen" the food journal proclaims (2004, 7).

If we are to go one step further, we can also generalize that among those who cook, there is a desire to feel knowledgeable, capable, and confident in the kitchen. The manifestation of this desire looks and feels different depending on the individual. To some, it is the idea of thrusting open the refrigerator doors after work, scanning the contents within, and effortlessly whipping together dinner for four. To others, it looks like a social gathering in which one can speak or edify extemporaneously on a culinary method or technique. To me, confidence and know-how present themselves in the form of my mother's kitchen, where there seemed to always be a large pot of anchovy- or beef-based stock set to a simmer that served as the base of any number of Korean soups or stews. Her kitchen spoke of continuity and cohesion, in which a company of ingredients and recipe components furnished one meal after another. My own, rather capricious, kitchen, in which I might make Thai beef and basil one night, pappardelle Bolognese the next, and roasted chicken with shallots the day after, lacks this sense of fluidity *and* manages to feel tired and monotonous at times.

With these basic observations in mind, we can evaluate the asynchronous resources and tools we turn to for everyday guidance and assistance based on how effectively they lead learners toward aptitude. One such category of resources are high-tech, low-touch technologies and innovations such as digital kitchen assistants and meal kits. By eliminating the need for meal planning or grocery shopping, conducting inventory of our refrigerators, or detecting the interior temperature of smoked meats and alerting us via smartphone of their doneness, these tools minimize human error by minimizing human involvement. The market demand for products and services such as these is high because they speak to a salient and persistent pain point: the work of feeding oneself and often others is unrelenting. But unlike ready-made meals and food delivery services, smart technology applications and cooking kits frame the act of cooking as desirable or identity-reinforcing. They are somewhat of a GPS navigation system for the kitchen, with an implicit message that the journey can be enjoyable once the burden of having to think too much or worry about failure is removed.

On the other side of the kitchen are high-touch, low-tech forms of guidance: conventional recipes and the media through which we encounter them (cookbooks, magazines, blogs, food shows, etc.). If their aforementioned high-tech cousins promise to remove the need for intuition, the members of this category exude it. Of utmost appeal, discerned through confident and descriptive language paired with impeccably casual imagery that holds as the current standard for content, is the embodiment of knowledge. Nikita Richardson of *New York Times Cooking* writes that the best cooking guides are "each a testament to the exciting-if-you-let-it-be art of cooking at home . . . while promising a glimpse of the cooks we can be if we just crack open the right book" (2021). The obvious benefit of detailed recipes is dissemination. In theory, anyone who is curious about any cuisine, chef, diet, ingredient, or method has an abundance of resources they can turn to. The disadvantage of detailed recipes is that they can be prescriptive and, relative to in-person learning, significantly more challenging to soak up knowledge from, as further discussed below. Nowadays it is common to see experts address these problems by offering alternative approaches to gaining expertise, such as *New York Times* food editor Sam Sifton's series of "No-Recipe Recipes" in which he encourages improvisation and adaptation beyond the confines of detailed instructions.

What both categories of resources lack is true comprehension of the mental load of novice cooks and the barriers to know-how. High-tech tools claim to take the hassle out of cooking, yet they overlook agency and the satisfaction of progress and growth. Aspirational cookbooks and food media destinations portray knowledge as within the learner's reach, without recognizing or addressing how a dizzying glut of content and the challenges of deciphering language into actions might impede one's ability to absorb information. This is not to say that these tools are without their merits (I own many of them) or that achieving knowledge through them is not possible (it is easier for some than others). Rather, it is to say that without appropriate scaffolding, home cooks are at risk of performing actions devoid of meaning, context, and connection.

In the field of cognitive psychology, the idea of "chunking" refers to a human being's tendency to group together sequences of thoughts or actions and transform them into automatic routines (Graybiel 1998). Behavioral chunks begin forming in infancy and alleviate the mental work of conducting complex tasks by turning them into second-nature embodied activities, such as walking or reversing a car out of the driveway. They speak to the importance of routinization and ontological security in that continuity and order enable us to function and advance in the world. If we follow instructions without an evolving framework for how and why the parts compose the whole, complex actions remain complex actions, which is exhausting. This, I believe, is the underlying frustration and sentiment among home cooks who lack a sense of foundation onto which they can build.

How to Know How

"Say something charming and funny," Eli instructed as my hands made a "magical pass" over a deck of cards. He was an undergraduate and the president of the NYU Magic Club, and I was a second-year doctoral student conducting a research project with my classmate Amy Wong for Bambi Schieffelin's Acquisition of Cultural Practices course in the Department of Anthropology. The assignment was to explore the transfer and co-construction of knowledge within a community of practice against themes we had covered over the semester: the structures of social action, framework analysis, language socialization, contextualization, and so on. Eli and I were both being videorecorded—he as the proficient, I as the novice—as he guided me through three magic tricks. I had approached the lesson focused on the physical mechanics of the tricks but found the performative aspects embarrassing and superfluous. So when Eli told me to say something charming and funny, I responded sardonically and self-consciously: "'Charming and funny.'"

What I failed to appreciate until Amy and I studied the tape later was that these seemingly excessive productions are strategic mis-directive techniques that speak to the credibility of "doing" magic. The singular goal of doing magic is to create an illusion that seems to have no logical explanation. As crucial as the mechanics of the trick are to its success, so too is the magician's ability to manipulate the audience's visual and commonsense understanding of the acts being performed. Verbal routines, gestures such as snapping fingers and blowing on cards, and other forms of embellishment are used as careful tools to structure a performance and steer the audience's attention. The magician consistently highlights mundane and irrelevant aspects of the trick while downplaying or obscuring moments in which sleight of hand is occurring. What Eli was beginning to show me was the critical value of having a verbal repertoire or a way of phrasing language to subtly guide the audience and shape the context of the trick's performance.

Learning to cook may not (always) require the same sort of flourish and performative demands as learning to do magic. Both, however, are part of disciplines that engage the material world, and both contain social worlds that are composed of rules, taxonomy, and knowledge that people share (or that *some* people share). I had excavated this research project and its corresponding notes from old digital archives because I remembered that Amy and I had detailed in it a macro-level process of teaching and learning that might have broader applications to knowledge formation. For one, the scaffolding we observed followed a cyclical and continuous pattern of demonstration-deconstruction-reconstruction-improvement. The proficient demonstrates and deconstructs an action (Eli shows me a step in the trick, then breaks down its movements), the novice observes and attempts to reconstruct the action (I mirror and reproduce Eli's movements), and the proficient and novice collaborate on improving said action (Eli provides feedback and makes adjustments, I ask questions and seek clarification on key features). The proficient structures the lessons in such a way that the novice gains more and more independence, speaking to Lev Vygotsky's concept of the *zone of proximal development* (Cole 1985, 155).

In parallel with cognitive scaffolding, however, is how the proficient shares the social dimensions of a practice through the articulation of beliefs, norms, and behaviors integral to a discipline (Webster 2003). Doing magic is as much about facility with existing mis-directive devices developed within the magic community that play on recognizable social and cultural patterns as it is physical dexterity. By modeling forms of embellishment, obfuscation, and lexical tools, Eli was invoking "organizational patterns that have an existence that extends far beyond the local encounter" (Goodwin and Duranti 1992, 2). Inasmuch as knowledge results from the combination of grasping experience and transforming it (Kolb 1984, 41), it is participation within and contribution to communities of practice that "directly penetrate actors to shape their habits and skills" in interaction with materials (Swidler 2001, 6). All this is to say that we metabolize information better when both cognitive scaffolding and social processes and contexts are synergistically attended to.

Authors Jean Lave and Etienne Wenger expand on this process of internalization by framing learning as a situated activity that takes place within a participation framework rather than the isolated mind. Knowledge, they observe through different apprenticeship communities in *Situated Learning: Legitimate Peripheral Participation* (1991), is not largely cerebral, nor are learners passive recipients of knowledge that benefit from a dyadic take-and-receive style of instruction. Learners are agents and whole bodies that undergo changing perspectives and developing identities as they move toward full membership within a community of practice. Learners do not unproblematically assimilate to a body of knowledge; they negotiate and renegotiate their membership in relation to others through continuous and centripetal social co-participation.

The "whole body" approach to knowledge acquisition is particularly apt considering that cooking is a discipline that demands attention from our corporeal bodies. We learn to interpret the consistency of different types of doughs—whether they spring back at you or maintain the impressions of your fingertips before slowly and hypnotically returning to their original state. We detect the Maillard reaction by sight, the blooming of spices through smell, the heat of a pan through the decibel of a sizzle, and the doneness of pasta by its resistant give between our teeth. Through our knives we feel the surface of a cutting board and hear the sharpness or dullness of a blade as it slices through a bell pepper. Cooking, like magic, is a discipline that requires procedural knowledge (know-how and how-to, e.g., tying shoelaces, swinging a tennis racket, woodwork, painting), which is distinct from declarative knowledge (static information and facts, e.g., state capitals, human biology). Whereas declarative knowledge is well transmitted through language and text-based forms of instruction, procedural knowledge is not. It develops most effectively from visual guidance, repetition, the aforementioned cycle of demonstration-deconstruction-reconstruction-improvement, and dialogical interaction and social co-participation within a community of practice.

The quickest way to draw ire on an online internet forum—whether one is cooking from a recipe or assembling a DIY gaming console—is to ask questions that have already been addressed in the instructions. The response "RTFM," which stands for "read the fucking manual," appears more on technical sites than culinary ones but ultimately captures that same spirit of light moral shaming that exists across disciplines. While there is no shortage of lazy learners and obvious questions in the world, perhaps the deeper issue is that whenever procedural knowledge is treated as declarative knowledge, confusion and lack of confidence are not unexpected consequences. In other words, it is not so much the learner but the absence of differentiation between categories of knowledge and the optimal conditions that facilitate them that inhibits the absorption and resonance of information.

The Progress of Man and the Demands of Human Nature

Introduced by psychologist Mihaly Csikszentmihalyi in 1990, the concept of *flow* is a state of complete and total immersion within an activity that makes the passage of time feel nonexistent. It is as nourishing to the psyche as it is exhilarating to the mind in that in this state, one feels the fullest expression of agency in their own lives. In her provocative book *Reality Is Broken: Why Games Make Us Better and How They Can Change the World*, Jane McGonigal states that the most popular video games are as successful as they are because game designers have become increasingly knowledgeable in the art of facilitating flow. Video games present ample opportunities for freely chosen work with clear and actionable goals, visible feedback, and powerful narratives that convey purpose and meaning. Game developers, McGonigal says, "are actively transforming what was once an intuitive art of optimizing human experience into an applied science" and consequently "becoming the most talented and powerful happiness engineers on the planet" (2011, 38).

One does not have to be a gamer to recognize this feeling of being completely activated—a state of optimism and confidence that stands in direct contrast to boredom and ineptitude. McGonigal's argument is not that video games are the solution to life's dissatisfactions but that the principles of good video game design can be applied to other structures of everyday life. Well-designed games provide voluntary and satisfying work—tasks that contain enough friction to be challenging but not so much as to be unachievable, that connect us to others and to a larger and greater purpose beyond our own existence (49). When I shared these notes with my brother and avid gamer, Michael, a few years ago, he told me about an element of a popular game called *God of War* (2018) in which the protagonist, Kratos, and his young son, Atreus, proceed to the next stage of the game by crossing a river by boat. Kratos makes use of the two minutes of crossing time to impart to his son part of the mythology that drives the game's central storyline. The gamer does nothing but listen. "At the end of the two minutes, you're supposed to proceed to the next step of the game," Michael said to me, "but I really didn't want the story to end." (Later, my friend Don informed me that game designers build in these entrancing periods of storytelling to maintain continuity while the next stage of the game is loading.)

This begs the question: with similar resources, ingenuity, research, and attentiveness to human nature as that spent on video game design, could the delivery of recipes be as captivating, enlivening, transportive, and fulfilling for a wider range of home cooks as *World of Warcraft* is for its demographic audience? Recipes are wellsprings of narrative, history, and lore. They abound with subjective knowledge, are ripe for discourse and debate, stretch across numerous areas of study and are continuously iterated on and transmitted across generations and cultures. And at the same time, a quick Google search today for "best lasagna recipe" yields thirty-nine million results in 0.54 seconds. For every beloved or storied recipe, there are hundreds, if not thousands, in circulation that lack meaning, context, and joy. Countless cookbooks boast "Over 100 Recipes" as their subtitle or marketing sell, while AI-enabled systems such as IBM's Chef Watson and Sony's Gastronomy Flagship Project train proprietary algorithms to generate "millions" of ingredient combinations and recipes (*Business Insider* 2015; Wiggers 2022).

Given everything we know about knowledge acquisition, information distribution, and pioneering design, it is quite possible to imagine a new framework for recipes that emphasizes experience over quantity, for those desiring it. And while advancements in voice recognition, AI, computer vision, and data science might feel antithetical to the deeply human and most ancient practice of transforming raw materials into comestible pleasures, these technologies can be used in service (rather than in lieu) of our desires to be productive and expressive through food. They can assist in removing unnecessary obstacles, enable the organization of content and information in a way that speaks to the requirements of procedural knowledge, offer opportunities for emotional and social engagement that are entirely at the learner's pace, and provide real pathways for progress.

As we ruminate over possibilities in culinary guidance, it might be helpful to consider educational anthropologist Peter McLaren's distinctions between three pedagogical styles in the ritual of instruction: teacher-as-entertainer, teacher-as-hegemonic-overlord, and teacher-as-liminal-servant (1988). Whether it is due to their educational setting, lack of planning, or performative style, entertainers (or worse, propagandists) engage their audiences but fail to lead them toward critical, reflective, and independent thinking. Hegemonic overlords do not even spark any real emotion or enthusiasm in their instruction, passing information onto others "as though it were a tray of food under a cell door" (165). Liminal servants, on the other hand, structure their guidance and delivery to enable students to become "primary actors" in the pursuit of knowledge "characterized by intense involvement and participation" (ibid.).

In cooking, or any domain of practice involving the material world, the ideal liminal servant would be one that synthesizes declarative and procedural knowledge toward the enablement of structural knowledge. An "internal connectedness" and "integrative understanding," structural knowledge enables practitioners to solve domain problems by applying the knowledge of *what* to the knowledge of *how*. Whereas entertainers and hegemonic overlords treat learners as spectators who "assimilate knowledge *about* things," liminal servants deliver guidance on knowledge "*of* things in relation to other things (knowledge as lived experience)" (166). With structural knowledge, learners develop the capacity not only to carry out tasks but also to expand and iterate on them, act on imagination with substance, and give rise to ideas and innovations far beyond the ability of any proprietary algorithm or smart robot.

Closing Thoughts

During a particularly long drive from North Carolina to Virginia, my husband and I were chatting about what our next car should be when I abruptly turned to him and said, "Know what I haven't had in a long time? Gum!" From the driver's seat, he did a double-take in my direction and said, "Where did *that* come from?" A low rattle coming from the luggage in the trunk had reminded me of my cousin Eugene's rooftop cargo carrier, which made me think of his son's motion sickness and my recommendation to give him hard candy to suck on to ease his stomach on long car rides, which led to memories of falling asleep with chewing gum in my mouth as a teenager and basically perforating my molars.

Unchecked and underdeveloped, the tendency to see and speak in tangents can be seen as a frustrating conversational habit. In food studies, it may not be such a bad thing.

Much of the work I do now falls under the realm of ethnomethodology, a form of qualitative analysis that examines the methods that people use in routine, everyday life through verbal and nonverbal interaction. Research begins with the understanding that there is a predictable order in social life that is public, observable, and knowable. My approach to the study of knowledge acquisition involves documenting patterns and practices, conducting long-form semi-structured interviews, mapping out frameworks that speak to the habits and needs of learners, and evaluating these frameworks based on flexibility, user experience, and scalability (i.e., how well they apply to a broader number of recipe types and styles). Nearly a decade removed from the doctoral program and heavily entrenched in the challenge of a new startup, I suffer zero fantasies that my research is as rigorous as that of a seasoned ethnographer. At the same time, if there is any merit to my work, it is owed to having had the opportunity to cultivate tangential thinking within and outside of food studies. Like an alien collecting microorganisms from distant planets to observe how they grow in her native environment, I am still witnessing how these intersections of theoretical frameworks and disciplines continue to produce such remarkable fruit.

REFERENCES

Appadurai, Arjun. 1988. "How to Make A National Cuisine: Cookbooks In Contemporary India." *Comparative Studies in Society and History* 30 (1): 3–24.

Blizzard Entertainment. *World of Warcraft.* Blizzard Entertainment. Microsoft Windows, macOS. 2004.

Business Insider. 2022. "We Tested Three Intriguing Recipes from a Hot New Chef (That Isn't Human)." https://www.businessinsider.com/.

Cole, Michael. 1985. "The Zone of Proximal Development: Where Culture and Cognition Create Each Other." *Culture, Communication, and Cognition: Vygotskian Perspectives*, edited by James Wertsch, 146–61. Cambridge, UK: Cambridge University Press.

Csikszentmihalyi, Mihaly. 2008. *Flow: The Psychology of Optimal Experience.* New York: Harper Collins.

Goodwin, Charles, and Alessandro Duranti. 1992. "Rethinking Context: An Introduction." In *Rethinking Context: Language as an Interactive Phenomenon*, edited by Alessandro Duranti and Charles Goodwin, 1–42. Cambridge, UK: Cambridge University Press.

Graybiel, Ann M. 1998. "The Basal Ganglia and Chunking of Action Repertoires." *Neurobiology of Learning and Memory* 70, no. 1–2 (July): 119–36. https://doi.org/10.1006/nlme.1998.3843.

Fisher, M. F. K. 1983. *With Bold Knife and Fork*. New York: Paragon.

Jaffe, David. 2018. *God of War*. Santa Monica Studio. Playstation 4.

Kolb, David A. 1984. *Experiential Learning: Experience as the Source of Learning and Development*. New York: Prentice Hall.

Lave, Jean, and Étienne Wenger-Trayner. 1991. *Situated Learning: Legitimate Peripheral Participation*. Cambridge, UK: Cambridge University Press.

McGonigal, Jane. 2011. *Reality Is Broken: Why Games Make Us Better and How They Can Change the World*. New York: Penguin.

McLaren, Peter. 1988. "The Liminal Servant and the Ritual Roots of Critical Pedagogy." *Language Arts* 65, no. 2 (February): 164–79.

New York Times. "The Best Cookbooks of 2021." 2022. https://www.nytimes.com.

Perez, Sarah. 2019. "Amazon and Google Double Down on Hands-Free Recipes to Help Sell Their Smart Displays." *TechCrunch*, November 14. https://techcrunch.com.

Shapiro, Laura. 2005. *Something from the Oven: Reinventing Dinner in 1950s America*. New York: Penguin.

Swidler, Ann. 2005. *Talk of Love: How Culture Matters*. Chicago: University of Chicago Press.

Webster, Helena. 2003. "Facilitating Critically Reflective Learning: Excavating the Role of the Design Tutor in Architectural Education." *Art, Design & Communication in Higher Education* 2 (3): 101–11. doi:10.1386/adch.2.3.101/0.

Wiggers, Kyle. 2022. "Sony AI Launches the Gastronomy Flagship Project to Apply AI to Cooking." *VentureBeat*, December 14. https://venturebeat.com.

10

Design

Food, Ethnography, and Materiality

FABIO PARASECOLI

Theory, Practice, and Everything in Between

A widespread sense of rupture and crisis in our increasingly unsustainable food system is one of the reasons behind the growing presence of food at the forefront of debates in civil society. At the same time, food has become an important way for people to shape and express their identities, both at the individual and the collective level. For instance, purchasing choices, such as going to the farmers' market, deciding to eat organic, consuming natural wines instead of traditional ones, or occasionally splurging on artisanal cheese are all performances that allow people to define who they are to themselves and to others and how they want to express themselves in the world.

The interest in these issues has stimulated the emergence of food studies programs. Growing numbers of students are turning to them to acquire the specific knowledge and abilities they need to contribute positively to changing the food system. In our program at NYU, specifically, they can choose to focus on media and communication, policy and administration, or social entrepreneurship. Whatever their specific emphasis may be, our students often find themselves torn between the need to research, study, and analyze their domain of interest and the desire to actually intervene in it. They constantly try to balance the intellectual efforts to expand their education in an academically rigorous manner with their expectations to learn methods and skills that they can apply in their work lives. The need to find real-life applications for their pursues is further complicated by the constant tension between the critique of the food system, the desire to be professionally successful in it, and the enticements to compromise with the forces that dominate it, from the industry to government authorities, which students cannot avoid if they want to operate effectively in the reality that surrounds them. Students constantly have to negotiate different priorities and values, ranging from economic goals to political outlooks. If they are concerned about issues such as citizen participation, inequality, and environmental sustainability, they may find it difficult to operate in a culture that is geared toward expanding production and consumption, while continuing to consider food a source of pleasure and community building.

As a scholar, a researcher, and a member of the New York University food studies community, I have been reflecting about these frictions. In our field, we inevitably deal with and operate within complex systems in which interventions may have all sorts of unpredictable effects. Planners and designers refer to these matters as "wicked problems," issues that are challenging or impossible to fix once and for all because of partial awareness, often contradictory elements, and constantly shifting contexts. Difficult to pinpoint and define, wicked problems cannot be examined with the goal of identifying a single, definitive solution or a stopping point, and addressing one concern may cause unintended consequences in other aspects (Rittel and Webber 1973). The global food system is certainly one of the most pressing wicked problems of our age. Finding ways to study, understand, and at times intervene in it presents itself as an urgent task.

This is one of the reasons why in the past few years I have been integrating both my research and my applied work with methodologies and theoretical approaches developed within the discipline and the professional world of design and, in particular, the new and inherently transdisciplinary field of food design. As the now dormant Food Design North America, of which I was one of the founding members, stated in its launch document, food design "includes any action that can improve our relationship with food individually or collectively. These actions can relate to the design of food products, materials, practices, environments, systems, processes and experiences" (Food Design North America 2014). This description perfectly reflects the ebullient state of food design, an umbrella concept with which professionals from different backgrounds can identify. As the field is still in its initial phases, different actors give it varied interpretations in terms of practice and research, conceptualizing what they do, their methodologies, and their theoretical perspectives in vastly divergent ways (Parasecoli 2018). Overall, food design embraces practical and project-oriented approaches based on the integration of qualitative and quantitative methodologies, with the objective to operate real—and possibly tangible—interventions in complex food systems.

At the same time, I have been able to contribute to design projects through my training in the humanities and the social sciences; in particular, I have been integrating the knowledge deriving from food studies and the ethnographic methodologies that I have been applying in my own research projects with the result-focused perspectives that are prevalent in design. In this essay, after discussing the relevance of design in food systems, I will explore the potential synergies between food studies, design, and ethnography to generate new theoretical insights, provide practical tools to operate in the food system, and establish generative pedagogical approaches that can be effectively used in the classroom or in workshops. The recourse to design and ethnography—the former emphasizing materiality and embodiment, the latter focusing on meaning and reflected experience—could help food studies overcome the much debated split between research on food culture and food systems, between highlighting agency or structure (Alkon 2018).

Design and Food Systems

The structural problems that plague the food system, neither natural nor inevitable, are no longer hidden by the illusion of abundance for everybody. However, it is necessary to avoid any nostalgic or luddite attitude, while acknowledging that technological advancements have drastically reduced the number of people suffering from hunger. At the same time, the concentration on efficiency and larger outputs, together with the food industry's constant quest for higher profits, has caused troubles ranging from environmental degradation and compromised personal health to unchecked injustice and exploitation. Against this background, we are constantly forced to choose between alternative futures. As we seek changes or at least look for viable solutions for current and possibly imminent crises, food is also revealed to us as a design problem (Parasecoli and Halawa 2019). As the food system was not created by a central authority, it is not a well-oiled assemblage in which all the parts are arranged to fit perfectly with each other, toward a predetermined objective. It is more realistic and accurate to conceptualize it as a jumbled ensemble of nodes that expand in every direction and change all the time, responding to all kinds of stimuli and pressures. We realize that the parts that work poorly are often man-made, constituting bad design and failures of foresight or empathy.

For this reason, food has attracted the attention of designers, reflecting the ongoing shift in their discipline and their practice from mainly objects and spaces (graphic design, industrial design, furniture design, architecture) to experiences and interactions. This evolution came about thanks, in part, to the spread of personal computers among both professional and non-professional users. Suddenly, there was a very complex machine that needed to interface with humans; for designers, it was important not only to understand the physical design and the affordances it allowed but also to appreciate its interface, its usability, and the users' reactions and relationship to it. In the past few years, design has shown growing attention toward processes, services, and systems, invisible dimensions that still maintain a deep influence on the material. Building on these premises, many designers now embrace what is often referred to as "design thinking," an iterative, practice-based method to look for better future arrangements rather than just for solutions to specific problems. After defining and researching the issue at hand, practitioners are supposed to generate and consider many possible ideas and strategies that should then be prototyped and put to the test. Additional insights can be obtained from testing and used to further generate ideas. The process can be iterated in order to refine solutions and to select the best one for implementation, which can expand learning (Cross 2011).

Design approaches are flexible and intended to operate in open and evolving situations, with numerous interconnected elements, and where conflicts of values and goals arise between participants. Design is better equipped to deal with wicked problems—including the global food system—than other disciplines and professional practices. This is especially the case when design is informed by systemic thinking, which, as Pourdehnad, Wexler, and Wilson (2011) argue,

> replaces reductionism (the belief that everything can be reduced to individual parts), cause and effect (environment free theory of explanation),

and determinism (fatalism) with expansionism (the system can always be a sub-system of some larger system), producer-product (environment-full theory of explanation) and indeterminism (probabilistic thinking). Additionally, it replaces analysis (gaining knowledge of the system by understanding its parts) with synthesis (explaining the role of the system in the larger system of which it is a part) (3).

As Ryan (2014) observes, "systemic design allows groups to appreciate situations from multiple scales and perspectives. It provides ways of deeply empathizing with stakeholders while working alongside them to collectively apprehend and construct a broader context within which to situate our challenges. Systemic design helps groups challenge boundaries, construct shared frames of reference, visualize alternatives to prevailing paradigms, and align actions to improve messy situations" (3).

Applying such principles, designers can participate in the development of projects that recognize and integrate the priorities, values, and needs of as many stakeholders as possible, especially those whose voices are less heard. Stakeholders arc no longer considered only as recipients of professional interventions by designers but rather as co-designers and participants. In the words of Ezio Manzini, designers "find themselves in a world where everybody designs and where . . . their task tends to be to use their own initiatives to help a variegated array of social actors to design better" (Manzini 2012, 2). Decisions, no longer left to the designers only, become instead part of larger debates and negotiations, generating new forms of participation and discussion. Who decides what needs to be designed, who identifies what's important, who defines the priorities? And how to prioritize priorities? How to make priorities become reality? All design is political if we look at it as a project-oriented approach to get from the present to a desired future. Design can be considered a form of future making (Yelavich and Adams 2014). Emotional and material elements need to be considered, and the negotiations with all the stakeholders involved may require time and effort. Of course, not all designers agree with these theoretical and methodological shifts, pointing out the risk for loss of specificity and skills that distinguishes professional designers from collaborators and amateurs.

The Challenges in Food Design

Design methodologies can support interventions in aspects of the food systems, in which material problems intersect with ideological and political issues. Connecting analysis with the generation of insights meant to guide action, design can strategically operate in many aspects of food systems at different scales, from the shape of a fork to the visual arrangement of a dining room, from the packaging of an industrial product to the structure and organization of a famers' market. Under the umbrella of food design, we find work ranging from culinary design and the study of the physical properties of food to the design of kitchen objects and appliances; technological innovations applied to growing, cooking, consuming, and disposing food; the reduction of kitchen and distribution waste; the organization of events and performances; the construction of permanent and temporary environments for food production, distribution, and consumption (artisan workshops, markets, restaurants, etc.); the management of services in hospitality and tourism; and food system strategies such as the organization of sustainable supply networks and the broadening of citizens' involvement in food-related issues.

Designers may respond to very diverse motivations and priorities, ranging from an alignment with the industrial food system to systemic interventions aimed at supporting local networks for production and consumption. They can contribute not only to the creation of new products, spaces, and experiences but also to making food production and distribution systems more equitable, efficient, and sustainable, balancing technological innovation with community needs and cultural priorities. Understandably, the food industry is often suspicious of design approaches whose explicit goal is to usher tangible—and possibly profound—behavioral changes among consumers. When the ultimate goal is to increase production and sales, corporations tend to favor projects in packaging, product design, graphic design, and to a more limited extent events, performances, and exhibitions, as long as these interventions support the introduction of new goods that can augment revenues without affecting the overall system and the structures that support it. However, large food businesses, especially if globally visible and vulnerable to criticism, are increasingly collaborating with food designers to rethink not only products, production choices, and supply chains but also their approach in terms of overall philosophy, sustainability, and involvement with the public.

This is a fundamental issue that many food designers face at some point: Is it possible to generate true innovation through partnership with food businesses, or is it instead necessary to create new spaces, parallel or alternative to the current corporate organizations? Food designers increasingly find themselves mediating among divergent worldviews and practices concerning the production and consumption of food, the individual and communal experiences that emerge from them, and their impact on larger issues such as sustainability, social justice, and public health.

Ethnography: Connecting Food Studies and Design

This last section will explore the potential synergies that can be established between food studies and food design, the visibility of which is growing in business, social entrepreneurship, the arts, performance, and to a lesser extent academia. I will then focus on ethnography and its methods as a possible bridge to connect the two fields, both theoretically and practically. Design, and in particular the new field of food design, can create and provide tools to develop approaches that can be effective to deal with the growing complexity of food systems. Partnerships between researchers and professionals in different fields contribute to this objective. Collaborative methodologies and practices can become more fruitful if they include food studies experts, with their analytical approach and their knowledge of cultures and food systems; designers, who are accustomed to working on concrete projects and to manufacturing and testing prototypes; and finally ethnographers, who have specific abilities to observe and understand the behaviors and inner worlds of everyone involved.

The analytical and critical tools developed in food studies can inform and integrate the practical applications that food design concentrates on. On the one hand, they can provide the necessary background information that would take a long time for designers to gather, even when their professional activities are dedicated to food. Food studies attention to cultural, social, economic, and political factors influencing the way we produce, distribute, consume, and dispose of food can shed light on the specific issues that designers may find themselves working on, allowing them to achieve important insights. This is particularly the case when food studies manage to overcome distinctions between sociocultural and systemic approaches, connecting structural and dynamic features of production networks and supply chains with the agency, choices, and values of all stakeholders involved.

At the same time, food design can help food studies scholars reflect on the applied potential and the implications of their work. Methodologically, designers often embrace abductive reasoning—observations that aim to identify the simplest and most plausible explanation for a phenomenon, even when at the moment it is not possible to positively verify it—as a methodology to deal with partial, shifting, and often contradictory data. Outlining "best available" or "most likely" theories can help proceeding with a more systematic inductive or deductive perspective, at times helping overcome the temporary lulls in research that may be fueled by self-doubt and excessive rumination. Furthermore, design methodologies such as design thinking and human-centered design provide pedagogical tools that can be successfully integrated in food studies, both in traditional academic courses and in intensive workshops, to teach students how to systematically reflect about specific issues in terms not only of analysis and assessment but also of the possible implementation of interventions, change, and innovation.

Ethnography can offer an important methodological link between food studies and food design. It supports researchers in shifting points of view, introducing greater empathy in the relationship with collaborators and interlocutors. It helps to understand the experiences, values, priorities, and goals of the stakeholders enmeshed in the food system, at all scales, while allowing those involved in a project to see problems and issues from different perspectives, which is essential to achieve original and creative ideas and insights. In doing so, ethnography questions common sense, revealing unexpected connections among stakeholders, invisible or under examined networks and assemblages of human and non-human actors, and emerging meanings, especially in research and practice projects focused on the experiential, the visual, and the sensory. Ethnography, as a participatory research method, does not allow looking at things from afar; ethnographers closely observe the phenomena they examine, in a granular and patient manner. This can also be done through virtual ethnographies of websites and social networks, which have become an important space for the development of individual and social identities and behaviors. These methodologies reveal food in everyday life as a network, system and a complex infrastructure in constant transformation; they remind us that culture is not only meanings and symbols but also objects and material practices.

Teaching and Researching at the Crossroad of Food, Ethnography, and Design

My engagement with design, and in particular with food design, is closely connected with my own academic path. Overall, my recent trajectory has moved from a purely theoretical kind of research to a more applied one, which engages with projects and concrete issues. When in 2010 I was hired at the New School, where I launched the undergraduate food studies program, I often found myself working with designers, as the bigger college of that university was Parsons, one of the most renowned design schools in the world. To be effective in that intellectual environment, it was almost inevitable that my research interests and my theoretical reflection shifted toward food design and to the relationship between food studies and design. I became a member of the first cohort of the Graduate Institute for Design, Ethnography, and Social Thought, which was meant to support faculty and graduate students in reflecting on the possible interactions across disciplines. This experience allowed me to take the time and think about food design, its present, and its future, while enhancing my familiarity with and practice of ethnography as a research method.

Collaborations with design scholars and practitioners have allowed me to be exposed to theories, methodologies, and practices—in particular human-centered design and design thinking—that I find complement the theoretical and analytical perspective of food studies, especially in endeavors centered on sustainability, justice, and social innovation. I participated in projects as diverse as the creation of workshops with the Red Cross Red Crescent Climate Centre to help people—in particular farmers—understand the complex connections between agriculture and climate change, or the exploration of new forms of more conscious, sustainable, millennial-friendly forms of chocolate consumption for a large international chocolate brand. I soon realized that my knowledge, built over years of research on food and food systems, could have practical applications, with all the tensions, contradictions, and negotiations they entail.

In the past few years, I have been interacting with food designers around the globe, both to better understand the field from a theoretical point of view and to operate in it. I am now involved with networks such as the International Food Design Society, Food Design North America, and the Red Latinoamericana de Food Design. I have also been supporting the efforts to launch a European association and collaborating with Food Design for Education (FDxE), an international group of scholars and instructors who are reflecting on pedagogy in the field.

Since I moved to NYU in January 2018, I have been looking for venues to expand my food design research, practice, and teaching. Besides launching a course focusing on food and design, I have introduced elements of food design and ethnographic research—together with more general reflections about materiality, visual cultures, and embodiment—in the Food and Culture graduate course. I prompted and guided students in doing interviews, observations, visual ethnographies, and digital ethnographies, with a particular focus on the physical environments in which food is produced, sold, and consumed. What does it mean to interview? How do you do it? What do you do with the information you get out of interviews? I teach them about content analysis and how to extract information from interviews. I also use observations, participant observations, and visual ethnography to help students better understand the material aspects connected with food culture and food systems, from objects to architecture and urban design. Through digital ethnographies, I push them to look at how communities and the discourses that support them develop online and in other virtual environments and how they affect other aspects of reality. What kinds of conversations happen on social media? What sort of words and framework of analysis are they using? What images do they produce? What are the ideas, the values, and the behaviors underlying those words and those images? These questions are also central in workshops that I have been developing in Denmark, Italy, Spain, Portugal, and the United States. The workshops, built around actual clients or specific aspects of the food system, have the goal of providing basic ethnography skills to students. At the end of the workshop, after gathering data through observation, interviews, and other ethnographic methodologies, students were able to pinpoint specific aspects that they thought could be changed or improved and to identify elements that could be introduced as new. At the same time, they were able to better understand their biases, values, and priorities, achieving a higher level of self-awareness.

In terms of research, I launched a long-term research project with Polish design researcher Mateusz Halawa we called "Global Brooklyn", focusing on a specific style of restaurant and café that has become popular around the world, especially among millennials. Its heavily postindustrial look and feel reflects a preference for repurposed material—reclaimed wood, rusty iron, exposed beams, and visible infrastructural elements. It embodies nostalgia for a less virtual world through menus in whimsical fonts on blackboards, Edison bulbs as lighting elements, mason jars as containers for drinks, and a certain preference for the analog over the digital. The research project, first outlined in an article (Halawa and Parasecoli 2019) and later developed into an edited volume (Parasecoli and Halawa 2021), is meant to build interdisciplinary connections between food studies, design, and ethnography, thanks to contributors from locations as diverse as Bogota, Mumbai, and Tel Aviv with different backgrounds and different professional experiences. The emerging aesthetic regime of Global Brooklyn aligns with powerful socioeconomic processes ranging from postindustrialization and gentrification of cities, struggles around justice and sustainability in the food system, to the rise of the digital.

This research project shows how food studies can engage—and should engage more—with the materiality of objects and constructed environments surrounding food and how they interact, shape, and reflect embodied experiences, memory, identity, culture, and the social relations built. The study of sensoria and the qualia that characterize them from a design point of view can draw greater attention to the impact that tools and technologies have on the way we relate to food, providing a new lens to observe familiar activities such as cooking and further eroding the distinction between subjects and objects, spirit and matter, which has already been the target of critique in food studies. The use of ethnography as a method bridging food studies and design can generate a better understanding of the complex relationship between materiality and affect, between the utility of objects and their meaning in practice.

I am also using design as an intentional and future-making approach in my research project with Mateusz Halawa and Agata Bachórz from Gdańsk University on the revaluation of regional and traditional food in Poland, based on a three-year grant from the National Science Centre, Poland. We noticed that many cultural intermediaries and tastemakers who are involved with this new approach to Polish food show designerly attitudes. They do not consider themselves designers, of course, because they are journalists, food producers, chefs, and entrepreneurs, but they operate like designers as they bridge the gap between the present and a desired future in an intentional way. They innovate by transforming materialities, creating new social and market connections and value chains, and by storytelling. Their practices are designerly because design is a mode of action where thinking and doing, or head and hand, are collapsed into one, because these practices are reflective, intentional, and knowledge intensive and because ideas appear in the world as material prototypes, be it a dish, a pop-up, an event, or a start-up, that are tested, refined, and reissued in engagement with the public. We are also trying to use design-thinking elements and approaches to lead workshops as a method to get ethnographic data for our research. In January 2019, for instance, we invited eight young Polish chefs between twenty-five and thirty-five years of age to the Polish Academy of Science. In a more conventional group discussion, we could have asked them, "What do you think about Polish food?" or "What do you think is happening now?" But we decided to understand how they imagine themselves in the future and how they want to get there. We had them work as if in a design studio, thinking about concepts, visions, and projects. We did not ask them to tell us what they thought but rather to create a menu for 2030.

In June 2023, thanks to a grant from the Ministry of Culture and Sports of Spain, I organized a two-day workshop at NYU Madrid, together with cultural management practitioner Gloria Rodriguez, during which designers and local food experts from public administrations and producers' associations reflected on possible approaches to raise the international profile of Spanish gastronomic heritage. Applying participatory design and cocreation methods, the participants were able to address the political tensions underlying all conversations about cultural and material heritage in Spain, as linguistic communities and autonomist movements question the national project as such. By doing so, they were able to take the first steps to develop a new, more inclusive framework to promote Spanish food that highlights shared practices and know-how rather than localized products and dishes. Although it was a pilot project, the workshop suggested that design methods have the potential to address the "wicked problem" of the political contrasts within food systems.

Reflections for the Future

The "wicked" nature of the problems plaguing the food system, resulting from complex and shifting factors ranging from biology to culture and from economics to politics begs for multidisciplinary—and possibly transdisciplinary—teamwork. Closer interactions between food studies researchers and food designers have the potential to tackle these issues efficiently, creatively, and fruitfully, although without any illusion and hubris about finding ultimate solutions to solve the big problems of the world. There is plenty of room for collaborations, small and big. Food studies can offer a unique contribution to food design education. The acquisition of critical thinking tools and analytical skills borrowed from history, anthropology, sociology, politics, economics, and media— just to mention some of the areas explored in food studies—can provide food design students and practitioners with fresh perspectives and more refined tools to develop their projects and interventions. Of course, food design education could directly incorporate elements and methodology from those disciplines, in particular anthropology (ethnography) and sociology (surveys and focus groups). However, food studies, with its accurate exploration of foodways and food systems, can offer focused, multifaceted, and accessible insights for designers to delve more effectively in food-related projects.

The collaboration between food studies and food design cannot be unidirectional. Design, with its unique theoretical tools, methodologies, and operational approaches that go beyond creating objects and spaces to focus on services and systems has the potential to play a growing role in reshaping food systems (Brown 2009). From a pedagogical point of view, by familiarizing themselves with design, food studies students can acquire a new set of tools that integrate their learning process with practice and help them bring their reflection from theory and analysis to possible applications. Furthermore, design and its applications in food design can teach food studies students how to develop applied projects, identify priorities, and manage strategies. These are low-hanging fruits that only require open-mindedness and desire to collaborate.

REFERENCES

Alkon, Alison Hope. 2018. "From Companion Planting to Cross-Pollination: Thoughts on the Future of Food Studies." Plenary Address. *Graduate Journal of Food Studies* 5, no. 2 (December).

Brown, Tim. 2009. *Change by Design: How Thinking Transforms Organizations and Inspires Innovation*. New York: Harper Business.

Cross, Nigel. 2011. *Design Thinking: Understanding How Designers Think and Work*. Oxford: Berg.

Food Design North America. 2014. "FDNA founding document." http://www.fdna.org/.

Halawa, Mateusz, and Fabio Parasecoli. 2019. "Eating and Drinking in Global Brooklyn." *Food, Culture & Society* 22, no. 19 (June): 4, 387–406. doi: 10.1080/15528014.2019.1620587.

Manzini, Ezio. 2015. *Design, When Everybody Designs: An Introduction to Design for Social Innovation*. Cambridge, MA: MIT Press.

Parasecoli, Fabio. 2017. "Food, Research, Design: What Can Food Studies Bring to Food Design Education?" *International Journal of Food Design*, 2, no. 1 (April): 15–25. doi: 10.1386/ijfd.2.1.15_1.

———. 2018. "Food, Design, Innovation: From Professional Specialization to Citizens' Involvement." In *Handbook of Food and Popular Culture*, edited by Kathleen Lebesco and Peter Naccarato, 27–39. London: Bloomsbury.

Parasecoli, Fabio, and Mateusz Halawa. 2019. "Rethinking the Global Table: Food Design as Future Making." In *Food: Bigger than the Plate*, edited by May Rosenthal and Catherine Flood, 80–89. London: Victoria and Albert Museum.

———. 2021. Global Brooklyn: Designing Food Experiences in World Cities. London: Bloomsbury.

Pourdehnad, John, Erica Wexler, and Dennis Wilson. 2011. "Systems & Design Thinking: A Conceptual Framework for Their Integration." *Proceedings of the 55th Annual Meeting of the International Society for the Systems Sciences-2011* 55, no. 1.

Rittel, Horst W. J., and Melvin M. Webber. 1973. "Dilemmas in a General Theory of Planning." *Policy Sciences*. 4 (2): 155–69. doi:10.1007/bf01405730.

Ryan, Alex J. 2014. "A Framework for Systemic Design." *form akademisk* 7 (4): 1–14. doi: 10.7577/formakademisk.787.

Yelavich, Susan, and Barbara Adams, eds. 2014. *Design as Future-Making*. London: Bloomsbury.

11

Network Science

Sugar in Contemporary Colombia

JUAN C. S. HERRERA

Academic disciplines allow us to approach the world using different theories, methods, and points of view. As a food studies scholar, my thinking has been shaped by a network science approach. I argue that by using network science, one can truly understand the complexities of food systems and food consumption as relational entities in which many parts are linked to each other. In this book chapter, I study the development of sweeteners in food recipes from Colombia from 1977 to 2017. The results show the relative importance of sugar over most of the period of study until the last decade, when the use of substitutes such as honey began to increase. This chapter aims to show the potential of network science for food studies by analyzing these ingredients that are essential to Colombia's recipes, food consumption, exports, and culture. This study is closely linked to my academic trajectory and reveals how the food studies program at New York University has shaped my thinking and the future direction of my research.

Sweeteners in Colombia

I cannot recall the first time I tasted sugar, but I can come up with a long list of sweet dishes that have been part of my life story and that carry significant cultural meaning. Whenever I have the opportunity to go to Colombia, my home country, I strive to find *merengón*, a dessert made by layering thin sheets of meringue, fruits, and whipped cream, traditionally sold from the back of parked cars on busy highways that connect cities with the countryside. This dessert is so popular in Colombia that it has recently been embraced by McDonald's in their line of McFlurries.

Other sweet delicacies that I long for are *cocadas* (an Afro-Colombian dessert with many variations but essentially made with coconut, nuts, and sugar), *brevas con arequipe* (figs boiled in syrup and filled with dulce de leche), *chocoramos, chokis, caballeros pobres* (sweet plantains filled with cheese and guava paste), *empanadas de ratón*, (cheese empanadas sprinkled with sugar), pork ribs in sugarloaf (non-centrifugated brown sugar) sauce, among other sweetened foods that are produced in traditional and industrial forms and are part of the diverse repertoire of Colombian dishes. My fondness for sweetened foods is closely linked to the historical, economic, political, and cultural background of Colombia.

When I grew up in Colombia, I dreamed of Snickers chocolates, M&Ms, and other sweets that were the most prized gifts one could get when someone returned from traveling overseas. This repertoire of imported sweet foods slowly joined Colombia's traditional indigenous dishes after 1991, when President César Gaviria's free market *apertura* policies transformed Colombia into an open economy. The availability of sweet foods and sweeteners changed as a panoply of imported foods transformed the way Colombians ate. As I grew up in Colombia, I witnessed this transformation, particularly after 2012, when Colombia signed a free trade agreement with the United States, Colombia's largest economic partner as of 2020 (World Bank 2020).

Along with the increase of available sweet foods in supermarkets, street vendor stalls, and other highly convenient locations, the Colombian food scene changed as it embraced local and global ideas. These ideas are linked to a broader sociocultural context that was embedded as the political and economics landscape changed.

The first of these ideas is the revaluation of Colombian dishes as young chefs, some of them trained abroad, embraced the diversity of the Colombian food system and food culture and sought to create the New Colombian Cuisine (Mahecha 2017). The second one is the growing awareness of the connection between heath and food consumption as obesity rates have grown considerably over the past decades, from less than 5 percent of the male adult population in 1976 to 17 percent in 2017 (Trading Economics 2020) and from less than 10 percent to 26 percent for the adult female population, respectively. The most notable example of this is the debate in the Colombian senate in 2016 in which there was a proposed soda tax that did not succeed (Vecino-Ortiz and Arroyo-Ariza 2018). Furthermore, associations and NGO's such as Red-Papaz (parents association) (Papaz 2020) are aware of the consequences of sugar consumption in noncommunicable diseases and health.

Another important political context that shaped how chefs embraced local cuisine was the peace agreement between the Colombian government and the FARC in 2015. The agreement proposed a "system for the progressive realisation of the right to food" (Colombia, National Government—FARC, Santos, and Jiménez 2016, 111). This system is to be implemented through "campaigns designed to promote the production and consumption of highly nutritious foodstuffs, the proper handling of food and the adoption of good eating habits, which will take territorial characteristics into account and promote the production and consumption of Colombian foods" (ibid., 33) among other initiatives that stress the importance of sustainable, organic, and "culturally appropriate" food and food security for accomplishing a "stable and lasting peace."

As I grew up in Colombia witnessing and living through these changes, I became passionate about understanding them. I longed to study their consequences by using a multidisciplinary approach that incorporates larger economic, social, cultural, and political contexts. This was the motivation to pursue a PhD in food studies at New York University and leave behind a career in banking as a credit risk analyst and my work for the Colombian president's office as a quantitative researcher in the reintegration process of ex-combatants from paramilitary and guerrilla groups. Understanding food culture in Colombia and studying its importance, how it helped shape the nation, and the way we perceived our food system and culture as food consumption became my passion.

To approximate food consumption and food culture in Colombia, particularly sweets, I use food recipes as my primary source of information. Although recipes do not necessarily reflect what a group of people eat—since they can be biased and aspirational and there is no way to track whether the recipes were actually cooked—they do provide important evidence that cannot be found in other primary sources. Examples of this evidence are lists of ingredients, preparations, ingredient combinations, quantities, images, and accompanying text that compose food recipes and can be used to understand food consumption and food culture (Albala 2012; Cusack 2000; Krohn 2013).

My research utilizes self-collected archival recipes from Colombia spanning forty years from 1977 to 2017 to explore how food preferences and consumption changed over the last decades. Since I have collected 5,981 recipes encompassing 557 unique ingredients, I use quantitative methodologies to study them. The main methodological approach I use is network science. The following section presents a brief overview of the network science of food recipes.

Methodological Approach: Network Science: Disentangling the Complexity of Food

Food is one of the most interconnected systems ever created by humankind. Each dish we consume contains one or more ingredients and is brought to us through an intricate web of links connecting the ingredients in the dish to the places where they come from. Similarly, the dish, which can be stored as a recipe, is a system in itself, as ingredients are transformed through preparation techniques to accomplish the final culinary whole. The combination of ingredients in the form of a dish ensures that we get the varied diet necessary for our survival.

Network science allows us to study food recipes by assessing ingredients as nodes that are connected to other ingredients. To create a network of ingredients from a collection or corpus of recipes, one will have to identify each pair of ingredients in the corpus and count the total number of recipes in which they appear together. Afterward, one can simply draw each ingredient as a node and create links between them, including the count of recipes in which they appear together as information in these links. This count can be represented in many ways; one can either draw nodes closer to each other if they appear together in many recipes (like lines of gravitational force between two planets) or draw thicker or thinner node edges to indicate the relative frequency of their appearance as a pair. This process has to be done until all the possible pairwise combinations of ingredients have been exhausted. There are several software tools that facilitate this process, such as Python's NetworkX or R's Igraph and Statnet or user-friendly interphases such as Visone, Gephy, Cytoscape, and Pajeck.

Since my interest is in understanding how food recipes change over time, my corpus of recipes is chronological. Creating a network of recipes on a chronological dataset entails decisions on the periodicity of the count. This can be done, say, for the recipes that appear in one year and then appear the next, or one can do this for every decade or another number of years or simply by looking at the total corpus of recipes and thus covering all the years. This is the approach I use to analyze my corpus of recipes that I collected from *Revista Carrusel*, a Colombian magazine that has published recipes since its launch in 1977 until today.

Results: Sweeteners in Colombia 1977–2017

Network science visualization tools can present information on large datasets in a clear and understandable form as it focuses on the relations between different parts of a system by representing the entities that take part in the system as nodes and their relationships as edges. Network science studies of recipes have shown how ingredient combinations are related to the chemical compounds responsible for food aromas in western European and North American cuisines but not in Indian and East Asian cuisines (Ahn and Ahnert 2013; Ahn et al. 2011; Jain, NK, and Bagler 2015a, 2015b; Simas et al. 2017), have found efficient ways to search for recipes on websites (Wang et al. 2008), have linked geographical proximity to recipe similarity (Sajadmanesh et al. 2017; Wang et al. 2008), and modeled the evolution of food recipes (Jain and Bagler 2018; Kinouchi et al. 2008; Kikuchi, Kumano, and Kimura 2017) along with other applications (Bogojeska, Kalajdziski, and Kocarev 2016; Kazama et al. 2017; Trattner, Kusmierczyk, and Nørvåg 2019; Tuwani et al. 2019).

The following visualization (figure 1) shows the accumulated network of ingredients in a corpus of 5,981 Colombia recipes containing 557 unique ingredients. This visualization highlights sweeteners in the network of ingredients. As can be seen here, some sweeteners such as syrup, corn syrup, honey, sugarloaf, sugar, condensed milk, and brown sugar appear in the middle of the network, hence they are central in this collection of recipes. This means that they play an important role in Colombian recipes. In contrast, sweeteners such as agave syrup, artificial sweeteners, molasses, and maple syrup appear in the margins of the network, and thus are not as central. Another aspect to highlight in this visualization is the size of the nodes, as I have programmed the visualization to represent the node degree, that is, the number of

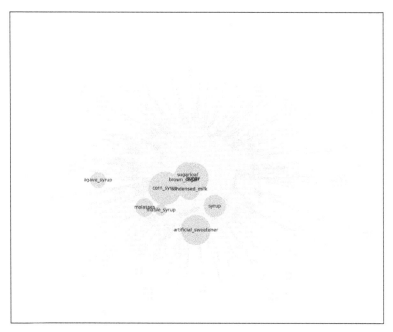

Figure 11.1: Sweeteners in a Colombian ingredient network, 1977–2017. The size of the nodes is relative to their degree, which is a measure of how important a node is in a network. Only nodes representing sweeteners have been highlighted and labeled. Total number of nodes: 557. This visualization was produced using Python's NetworkX and Mathplotlib

other ingredients to which each ingredient is connected. From a visual perspective, some sweeteners are more central than others in this network of ingredients, but we need a better definition of importance or centrality.

One of the most famous and more widely used statistical metrics for assessing the importance or centrality in a network is PageRank. This statistical measure devised by the founders of Google and presumably still powering the website "measures the relative importance of [a] webpage" (Page et al. 1999, 2), assigning a higher score to those that are more important and a lower score to those with lower importance. This process is accomplished by using algorithms that check how webpages are linked to each other, giving more importance to web pages that are linked to many others, particularly for those web pages that are linked to

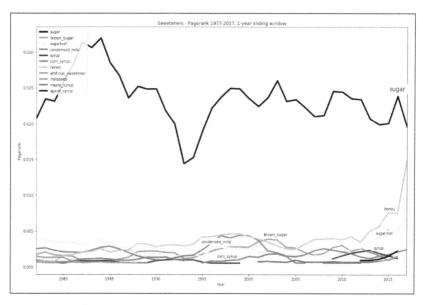

Figure 11.2: Yearly PageRank of sweeteners in a Colombian network of recipes 1977–2017 using a one-year sliding window. Each dot in the line represents the PageRank of each sweetener in a corpus of recipes published in a given year (for example, all the recipes published in 1977).

by more important web pages (Page et al. 1999). It is possible to use this statistic to study a network of ingredients in food recipes; however, this type of network is not as directional as the World Wide Web, in which web pages link *to* other web pages. In the ingredient network, ingredients are linked to others, but there is no directionality, hence I use a modified version from the original algorithm that still scores more important nodes higher to study the importance of sweeteners over time. Figures 2, 3, and 4, below, show the PageRank score for each sweetener in the corpus of recipes.

Each datapoint in the PageRank score in figure 2 has been calculated by creating a network for each year from 1977 to 2017 and computing the PageRank statistic for each year. For example, to compute the score for the year 2000, I created a network by taking into account all the recipes published in 2000 and counting the number of recipes in which each pair of ingredients appearing in that year's recipes appear together, and then I calculate the PageRank score of each ingredient. It can be seen in figure 2 that sugar was by far the most important sweetener during the whole period of study in this corpus of recipes. This is particularly salient for the period between 1977 and 1990. Afterward, its importance shows a notable decrease, which is picked up by honey. Nevertheless, sugar's importance grows after 1994 and remains relatively stable. It is more interesting to look at the role of honey and sugarloaf, which gained considerable traction after 2005.

In figure 3, one can see the importance of different sweeteners throughout the year to study seasonality, here demarcated by annual festivities (such as Christmas and Halloween), since Colombia's Equatorial location obviates the use of climactic seasonal phases. The PageRank score in figure 3 has been calculated by creating one network for each month of the year but aggregating the years (January, for example, contains all the recipes published in every first month of the year from 1977 to 2017, thus forty-one years). Figure 3 shows how the consumption of sugar peaks in December. It is also interesting to see how the beginning

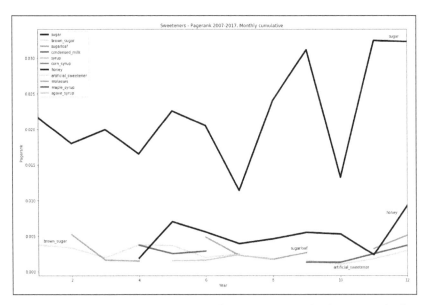

Figure 11.3: Monthly cumulative PageRank of sweeteners in a Colombian network of recipes 1977–2017. Each dot in the line represents the PageRank of each sweetener in a corpus of recipes published in the same calendar month over forty-one years (for example, all the recipes published in any January from 1977–2017).

of the year starts with lower consumption of sugar and grows slowly until December. This may indicate the importance of dieting after the beginning of a new year and indulgence around Christmas, which is marked by sweets such as *natilla* (sugarloaf pudding), sweet sauces for pork or turkey, Christmas confectionery, *manjar blanco* (rice pudding), *arroz con leche* (rice pudding), Christmas cake, and panettone.

Since aggregating the months of forty-one years may give a biased perspective, I built a network aggregating the months for each decade (figure 4). It is interesting to see how in the past two decades (lower row), notably in the past decade (lower right), October shows a peak in the importance of sugar as compared to earlier decades (upper row). This may be a result of Colombians' embrace of Halloween in recent decades. Along the lines of the yearly analysis, one can see how in the most recent decade (lower right), honey increases in importance.

As can be seen in these visualizations, sugar is a key ingredient in Colombian food consumption as approximated in recipes. While sugar is the most important ingredient according to PageRank, the results show that the importance of sugar has decreased in recent years. Perhaps due to debates on health and obesity, as Colombia's obesity rates have climbed, honey began to be positioned as a sugar alternative. This analysis, obtained using network science, allows me to understand the role of each ingredient over time and can inform a deeper inquiry of my recipe dataset using qualitative methods such as historical research by studying the sources and their content, particularly the text that accompanies the recipes.

Honey as a substitute for sugar has been touted in *Revista Carrusel* since 1984, in Ettica's piece *Sabor a Miel* (Honey's taste), which appeared along with five recipes using honey: "Honey is a natural and organic sweetener that has a distinctive flavor. . . . It is not aphrodisiac, it does not cure respiratory illness and it is not better tolerated by diabetics than sugar or other carbohydrates. . . . Generally you can use honey instead of sugar measure by measure, but in some baking and pastry recipes you need to be careful" (Ettica 1984). Hence, we know that honey was a known substitute for sugar, we can infer that Colombian folk medicine attributed some benefits to honey. The question is, Why wasn't honey as important in the past decade? I will now turn to my primary sources to look at the other pieces in the magazine that accompany sugar to see whether there has been a change in attitudes toward it.

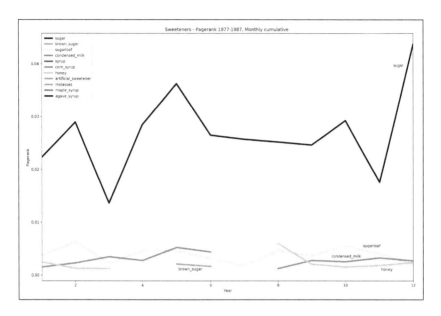

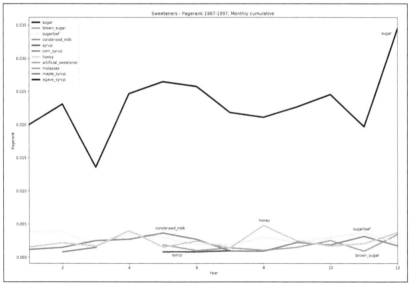

Figure 11.4: Monthly cumulative PageRank of sweeteners in a Colombian network of recipes 1977–2017. Each dot in the line represents the PageRank of each sweetener in a corpus of recipes published in the same calendar month over ten years. For example a dot in January represents the PageRank for 11.4.1 consisting of all the recipes published in any January from 1977–1987; 11.4.2 consists of all the recipes published in any January from 1988–1997 and so on.

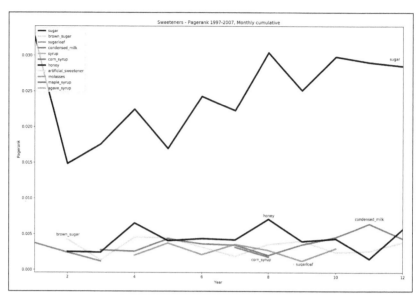

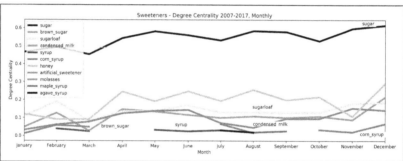

Figure 11.4: (Continued)

A *Revista Carrusel* reader's perception of sugar was influenced by the magazine's advertisements promoting sugar. For example, in 1996, Manuelita, one of the largest refined sugar companies in Colombia, took out a full page ad to explain how "pure, 100% natural, and healthy" (Manuelita 1996) sugar was obtained (figure 5), a particularly misplaced add since in the previous edition the magazine had run a piece on diabetes (November 1, 1996). Several other editions contain ads for condensed milk and sugar. The first piece on diabetes in *Revista Carrusel* appeared in 1985. This piece by Ettica titled "The Joy of Carbohydrates" touts whole "complex carbohydrates" as being associated with "lower incidence of diabetes, sclerosis, heart disease, and obesity" (Ettica 1985). Nine years passed until the next mention of diabetes in 1995, in another piece on fiber. It wasn't until the 2000s when several pieces on diabetes appeared, notably after 2005; probably the most informative one, from 2006, contains statistics on the incidence of diabetes in Colombia, noting that

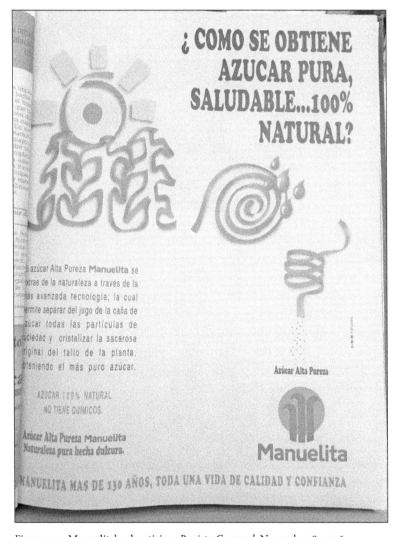

Figure 11.5: Manuelita's advertising. *Revista Carrusel*, November 8, 1996.

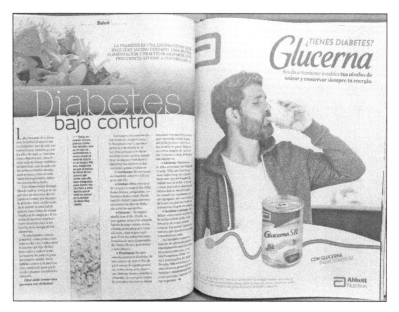

Figure 11.6: Glucerna's advertisement next to a piece on "Diabetes under Control," taken from *Revista Carrusel*, February 25, 2016.

2.2 million Colombians and thirty million Latin Americans have been diagnosed with the disease (*Revista Carrusel* 2016a). Additionally, the magazine contains advertisements for diabetes-related products such as the low-glycemic product line from Glucerna that appeared in 2016, conveniently located next to a piece entitled "Diabetes under Control" (*Revista Carrusel* 2016b) (figure 6).

This may be part of the explanation behind honey's ascendance in importance in the most recent decade along with broader debates on healthy eating.

Conclusion: Network Science and Food Studies

My interest in understanding changes in food consumption in developing countries by examining my own life story led me to join the food studies PhD program at NYU. During my PhD, I have studied statistical techniques in network science and econometrics, along with courses on social sciences and humanities. My approach takes a multidisciplinary stance that allows me to study large datasets of primary sources to gain an understanding of food consumption and food production using network science; this allows me to analyze large datasets and study them to find information that can be explained using qualitative techniques. The food studies program has provided me with a holistic approach to problems of food and culture and diverse methodological and theoretical tools to approach them.

Moving forward, I anticipate expanding my research in four ways. First, I am looking forward to connecting my professional and academic experience in both food systems research and conflict studies in Colombia by studying the relationship between conflicts, food security, changes in agrarian and fishing resources, and climate change to inform research in peace and stability in Colombia and the Andean region.

Second, I intend to link ingredient pairings with health, longevity, and wellness by researching color pairings in food dishes. Toward this aim, I expect to create a two-mode network in which colors are connected to dish names. Afterward, I plan to project this two-mode network into a one-mode network containing only color names. I hypothesize that healthier dishes (which can be measured using nutrition information from the USDA) are more colorful.

Third, I want to further my food studies research by modeling complex supply-chain systems that connect recipes, as an approximation of food consumption and food preferences, to gain a better understanding of organic agriculture and its relationship to urban consumers. I am particularly interested in studying this available data by modeling a supply chain using organic food producers, handlers, and supermarkets with geographical information systems and network analysis.

Fourth, my long-term vision is to establish a multidisciplinary research lab centered around understanding the complexities of sustainable food systems and conflict/peace using mixed-methods techniques. I expect that the outcomes of my research and that of my collaborators using network science, quantitative techniques, and regard for cultural preferences may inform food policy decisions that have a measurable impact on sustainability and human and environmental health.

Supplementary Materials

For the sake of conducting reproducible research, this text is accompanied with the code used to produce the findings. The code is hosted on https://github.com/juancsherrera/sweetnessandnetworks. The databases may be obtained by writing to the author at jsh501@nyu.edu for reproducibility purposes only and with a confidentiality agreement.

REFERENCES

Ahn, Yong-Yeol, and Sebastian Ahnert. 2013. "The Flavor Network." *Leonardo* 46, no. 3 (June): 272–73. https://doi.org/10.1162/LEON_a_00569.

Ahn, Yong-Yeol, Sebastian E. Ahnert, James P. Bagrow, and Albert-László Barabási. 2011. "Flavor Network and the Principles of Food Pairing." *Scientific Reports* 1, no. 196 (December). https://doi.org/10.1038/srep00196.

Albala, Ken. 2012. "Cookbooks as Historical Documents." In *The Oxford Handbook of Food History*, edited by Jeffrey M. Pilcher, 227–40. Oxford: New York: Oxford University Press.

Bogojeska, Aleksandra, Slobodan Kalajdziski, and Ljupco Kocarev. 2016. "Processing and Analysis of Macedonian Cuisine and Its Flavours by Using Online Recipes." In *ICT Innovations 2015: Emerging Technologies for Better Living*, edited by Suzana Loshkovska and Saso Koceski, 143–52. Berlin: Springer

Colombia, National Government—FARC, Juan Manuel Santos, and Timoleón Jiménez. 2016. "Final Agreement to End the Armed Conflict and Build a Stable and Lasting Peace." https://www.peaceagreements.org/viewmasterdocument/1845.

Cusack, Igor. 2000. "African Cuisines: Recipes for Nation-Building?" *Journal of African Cultural Studies* 13 (2): 207–25. https://doi.org/10.1080/713674313.

Ettica. 1984. "Sabor a Miel." *Revista Carrusel*, August 3.

———. 1985. "La Dicha de Los Carbohidratos." *Revista Carrusel*, June 21.

Jain, Anupam, and Ganesh Bagler. 2018. "Culinary Evolution Models for Indian Cuisines." *Physica A: Statistical Mechanics and Its Applications* 503:170–76.

Jain, Anupam, Rakhi NK, and Ganesh Bagler. 2015a. "Spices Form the Basis of Food Pairing in Indian Cuisine." *ArXiv:1502.03815 [Physics, q-Bio]*, February. http://arxiv.org/abs/1502.03815.

———. 2015b. "Analysis of Food Pairing in Regional Cuisines of India." *PLOS ONE* 10 (10): e0139539. https://doi.org/10.1371/journal.pone.0139539.

Kazama, Masahiro, Minami Sugimoto, Chizuru Hosokawa, Keisuke Matsushima, Lav R. Varshney, and Yoshiki Ishikawa. 2017. "Sukiyaki in French Style: A Novel System for Transformation of Dietary Patterns." *ArXiv Preprint ArXiv:1705.03487.*

Kikuchi, Y., M. Kumano, and M. Kimura. 2017. "Analyzing Dynamical Activities of Co-Occurrence Patterns for Cooking Ingredients." In *2017 IEEE International Conference on Data Mining Workshops (ICDMW)*, 17–24. https://doi.org/10.1109/ICDMW.2017.10.

Kinouchi, Osame, Rosa W Diez-Garcia, Adriano J Holanda, Pedro Zambianchi, and Antonio C Roque. 2008. "The Non-Equilibrium Nature of Culinary Evolution." *New Journal of Physics* 10 (7): 073020. doi 10.1088/1367-2630/10/7/073020.

Krohn, Deborah L. 2013. "Reflecting on Recipes." In *Cultural Histories of the Material World*, edited by Peter N. Miller, 226–32. Ann Arbor: University of Michigan Press.

Mahecha, Juliana. 2017. "A New Culinary Culture in Colombia: Equality and Identity in the Interpretation of Traditional Cuisines." PhD diss., Cornell University. https://ecommons.cornell.edu.

Manuelita. 1996. "Manuelita." *Revista Carrusel*, 6 November 6.

Page, Lawrence, Sergey Brin, Rajeev Motwani, and Terry Winograd. 1999. "The Page-Rank Citation Ranking: Bringing Order to the Web." Stanford InfoLab.

Red PaPaz. 2020. "Red Papaz—About." https://www.redpapaz.org/.

Revista Carrusel. 2016a. "Diabetes, un Azucar Amargo." April 21.

———. 2016b. "Diabetes under Control." November 6.

Sajadmanesh, Sina, Sina Jafarzadeh, Seyed Ali Ossia, Hamid R. Rabiee, Hamed Haddadi, Yelena Mejova, Mirco Musolesi, Emiliano De Cristofaro, and Gianluca Stringhini. 2017. "Kissing Cuisines: Exploring Worldwide Culinary Habits on the Web." In *Proceedings of the 26th International Conference on World Wide Web Companion*, 1013–21. Republic and Canton of Geneva, Switzerland: International World Wide Web Conferences Steering Committee. https://doi.org/10.1145/3041021.3055137.

Simas, Tiago, Michal Ficek, Albert Diaz-Guilera, Pere Obrador, and Pablo R. Rodriguez. 2017. "Food-Bridging: A New Network Construction to Unveil the Principles of Cooking." *ArXiv:1704.03330 [Physics]*, April. http://arxiv.org/abs/1704.03330.

Trading Economics. 2020. "Colombia—Prevalence of Obesity, Male (% Of Male Population Ages 18+)." 2020. https://tradingeconomics.com.

Trattner, Christoph, Tomasz Kusmierczyk, and Kjetil Nørvåg. 2019. "Investigating and Predicting Online Food Recipe Upload Behavior." *Information Processing & Management* 56, no. 3 (May): 654–73. https://doi.org/10.1016/j.ipm.2018.10.016.

Tuwani, Rudraksh, Nutan Sahoo, Navjot Singh, and Ganesh Bagler. 2019. "Computational Models for the Evolution of World Cuisines." *ArXiv Preprint ArXiv:1904.10138*.

Vecino-Ortiz, Andres I., and Daniel Arroyo-Ariza. 2018. "A Tax on Sugar Sweetened Beverages in Colombia: Estimating the Impact on Overweight and Obesity Prevalence across Socio Economic Levels." *Social Science & Medicine* 209: 111–16. doi: 10.1016/j.socscimed.2018.05.043.

Wang, Liping, Qing Li, Na Li, Guozhu Dong, and Yu Yang. 2008. "Substructure Similarity Measurement in Chinese Recipes." In *Proceedings of the 17th International Conference on World Wide Web*, 979–88. https://doi.org/10.1145/1367497.1367629.

World Bank. 2020. "Colombia Trade | Data." 2020. https://wits.worldbank.org/country snapshot/en/COL.

12

Library Sciences

A Bibliometric Perspective of "Food Studies"

JAMES EDWARD MALIN

Introduction: Craft in Research

Like many food studies peers, I once spent several years honing skills in a kitchen, behind a counter, and in front of a cutting board. I believed contentment lay on the other side of hours counted in calloused digits and charred ambitions. That with determination, my craft would amalgamate into the quiet confidence of ability. Unfortunately, I came to understand that for me, this goal was problematic. It took me years to discover that what I loved in the kitchen (and on the plate) was food's history, context, and significance. The craft of cooking and my appetite for understanding culinary culture never seemed to meet. In restaurants, there were always lucky happenstances—passing conversations of exotic techniques, a curiosity of how milk foamed differently in summer than in fall—but I never seemed to find a community interested in sharing knowledge, teaching, and learning about food. Indeed, I came to discover that in the food service industry, learning *about* food, *about* cooking, or *about* restaurants was severely subordinate to their actual execution. The goal, after all, in much of food service mastery is to turn one's brain *off*. For me, however, without understanding how, when, or why I was exercising my craft, I felt I had little direction.

My dreams were idyllic but not necessarily grandiose. I wanted fulfillment, not to be a star. For many aspirational chefs, the axiom of success was *chef de cuisine* in Escoffier's almighty brigade. The head chef position—white toque, notoriety, and artistry, with which came power, expression, and adulation. However, my longing and focus pointed toward a less sought-after position that I discovered one day while scouring my purposefully beat-up and jacket-less *Larousse Gastronomique*. *Chef communard* (or sometimes staff chef) was a position in the traditional company that cooked internal *family* meals for the workforce. This became my secret desire: to use a restaurant's leftovers and aging ingredients to covertly satiate the creators of cuisine. I wanted to work among chefs, but not on the line; I wanted to help nurture and bolster *their* craft.

Unfortunately, as I quickly discovered, *chef communard* was an aberration of the past. As it turned out, my dream existed only in books and history. Instead of giving up, however, I turned my career toward the books and history themselves. In 2016, I matriculated into the first cohort of a brand-new dual master's degree in food studies and library and information science. In this program, I trained as a librarian and learned how to support food research itself while studying food culture. Because of this, I feel that I have attained *chef communard*; as a librarian, I cook for the chefs, not the dining room—only the chefs are scholars, and their kitchen the library.

Why Is Food Studies Research So Hard?
A Librarian's Perspective

In some ways, I have learned that academic research is similar to cooking professionally; techniques take discipline to master, arcane traditions abound, and expediency and humility are paramount. Most of all, however, it is never over, never perfect, and never complete. Calluses and burns are certainly more challenging to come by in a library than in a kitchen, but late nights and endless coffees are not. While research in any discipline is challenging to master, food studies asks inquirers to learn research techniques in what might be comparable to *staging* in multiple restaurants all at once. Wading through its various canons and diverse methodologies is like trying to learn how to make the perfect tagliatelle in a ramen restaurant; everything is there, but you might end up with a different noodle.

This problem is often attributed to the multidisciplinary nature of the field. Multidisciplinarity is a theoretic style of cross-disciplinary academics, a concept that first gained popularity among science-ethicists in the 1970s but has since come to define something of a renaissance among liberal arts. According to Klein (2010), there are three cross-disciplinary typologies, which in addition to multidisciplinarity include interdisciplinary and transdisciplinary fields. Whereas interdisciplinarity seeks to manufacture an entirely new field with aspects of others (for example, how art history melds fine arts with history), and transdisciplinarity describes work that exclusively undergirds all fields (like critical theory), multidisciplinary fields are characterized by how they "juxtapose separate disciplinary approaches around a common interest, adding breadth of knowledge and approaches" (Klein 2015, 276). Within this category, food studies positions food as the common interest around which perspectival frames are attached from other, established disciplines. (Note that although several scholars I cite propose conflicting or complementary structural relationships of these concepts [Choi and Pak 2006; Gullbekk, Boyum, and Bystrom 2015; Huutoniemi et al. 2010], for this chapter, I adhere to Klein's definitions and taxonomy.)

Field barrier-breaking has a countercultural subtext, what Steve Fuller (2012) described as "deviant interdisciplinarity," and this feeling among the food studies community is well documented. Warren Belasco (2008) stated that although "food studies is now 'respectable,' it is also inherently subversive" (6). Lisa Heldke (2006) warns her students that to study food, "you had better be prepared to develop a thick skin" (202). On top of cultural polarization, cross-disciplines' nonconformity incur heavy institutional costs, evident in the shape of library support.

Cross-disciplinary fields are notoriously tricky to support bibliographically. Birger Hjørland (2005, 2009, 2011) and Hope A. Olson (2007) both have shown how their novel structures call for entirely new modes of information organization and, thus, radically different librarianship. Whereas Hjørland posited that conceptual domains are entirely new models of categorization, Olson showed how multidisciplinary vocabulary flatten organized hierarchies. (These break the usual Aristotelian framework that allows a librarian to point to *their* subject.) It is clear that academic cross-disciplinarity requires a new and messier model of information organization that does not fit with traditional paradigms.

The difficulty is attributable to the retrospective nature of organizing information and developing research services, both of which historically demanded relatively fixed goalposts to aim at. Cross-disciplinarity, however, is anything but stagnant. A cross-discipline may polarize and

fracture perspectives in one place or time and galvanize communities together at others. Astroff (2012) goes as far as to describe the push and pull
of disciplines and cross-disciplines as "culture wars" (11). Confusingly for
librarians, some cross-disciplines have such an impact that they have been
reabsorbed back into the forefront of their progenitors, or at the same
time distinguished themselves with their own additional departments
and programs. (For example, feminist studies and critical race studies are
notably difficult to locate within traditional academics.) Libraries' static
constraints (space, budgets, staff, and others) make it difficult to support
cross-disciplinary inventiveness and re-inventiveness. However, whereas
this issue was once inherent, today's minimized reliance on bookshelves,
card catalogs, and specialized ancillary collections can lessen the impact.

Unfortunately, although new digital research infrastructures have the
potential to revolutionize cross-disciplinarity, right now they instead use
anachronistic design approaches. As Larivière, Haustein, and Mongeon
(2015) showed, "The form of the scholarly journal was not changed by the
digital revolution. The PDF became the established format of electronic
journal articles, mimicking the print format" (2). The portable document format (PDF) has allowed publishers to mimic printing articles,
binding artificial volumes and issues, and even enumerating imitation
page numbers. (In this way, digital scholarly journals are skeuomorphic
in retaining design elements correlated with the function of their original printed form, even though they no longer need the design element's
original functionality.)

Even keyword searching in databases is a digital facsimile of index
research. To explain: when a scholarly article is published, it is cataloged
with a corresponding record representing various metadata like title, author, journal name, and others. These records are then bundled together
and sold as bibliographic databases. These record bundles are what
scholars probe to retrieve articles or information they seek—a digital
synonym of paging through journals, books, and bibliographies. Contemporary bibliographic academic research, therefore, is not querying a
vast full-text amalgam of knowledge for an idea or concept, as it may appear. In actuality, researchers are meant to use fixed fields and standardized terminology. Such controlled structures dictate specific points of
entry. One may search only through titles, for example, or search solely
within abstracts.

The systems that describe and index articles' content, however, are called *subject keywords*. (In different databases, these are referred to differently, as *keywords, index terms, subjects, standardized vocabulary, subject headings*, and others, but for consistency, I refer to them as *subject keywords* throughout this work.) These database vocabularies and their taxonomies develop through practice over time. Researchers get to know their discipline's subject keywords, while simultaneously, catalogers get to know what subject keywords are most useful to scholars. This closed, positive feedback loop creates what Marcia Bates (1996) described as "a cynosure of an extensive social and documentary infrastructure [in which] academic fields develop a common vocabulary and research style" (159). Nevertheless, this cooperation never works for cross-disciplinary fields, whose conceptual subjects originate from various disciplines and thus manifold vocabularies.

Without a common lexicon, food studies scholars "tend to overlook materials that are published in other fields" (Duran and MacDonald 2015, 234). Food studies departments, faculty members, researchers, and students may produce an enormous amount of published academic content each year, but no single or canonical forum (platform, database, website) exists for food studies conversations. This lack of cohesion frustrates many stakeholders in the field (Hamada et al. 2015; Nestle and McIntosh 2010). Furthermore, it makes the bar for entry high (Korr and Broussard 2005). A few attempts have been made to create a canonical platform (for example, Bloomsbury's Food Library or Alexander Street's Food Studies Online), but all have proved insufficient. That said, any attempt to make a comprehensive food studies research database (with, for example, standardized and controlled vocabulary) might seem to defeat the very purpose of multidisciplinary juxtaposition.

Instead of trying to fit cross-disciplinary pegs into disciplinary holes, librarians and food studies researchers alike require a new way to conceptualize cross-disciplinary bibliographic research. Food studies scholars need a way to understand what I describe as *cross-research*. One example of novel cross-research support might be to survey and map subject keywords that co-occur with food studies among the broadest-reaching, general peer-reviewed article databases in academia. (One may seek how different are the research vocabularies of, for example, food history from those of flavor chemistry? What words are shared, and what must be translated?) By studying the nuance of how food studies literature is organized, scholars should better understand the concepts that make up the domain. With this lexical topography, food studies researchers may more deliberately choose what search vocabulary will yield the best results for their respective disciplinary frame. (In what area of food studies, for example, do scholars use the word *diet* instead of *nutrition*?) Additionally, such a map could help scholars see where subjects overlap disciplines. (For example, the subject keyword *neoliberalism*, which most commonly occurs in the sociological part of the field, may be collocated with subject keywords like *social support* and *weight* in articles originating from dietetics journals.)

Mapping the Food Studies Domain

The rest of this work aims to answer a simple question: What does the moniker "food studies" mean across scholarly article research? To answer this question, I collected and mapped the subject keyword terminology assigned to relevant literature from several large databases. To search exhaustively across them and their vocabularies, I implemented an evidence synthesis (ES) methodology—a category of reproducible and procedural protocols commonly used among health librarians and informationists to exhaustively gather all evidence pertinent to a specific decision or recommendation (Cochrane 2004). Scoping reviews, for example, are an ES type used "to map the key concepts underpinning a research area, as well as to clarify working definitions, and/or the conceptual boundaries of a topic" (Peters et al. 2020). Proposed in 1999 (Hagell and Bourke Dowling 1999), scoping reviews were later given a framework (Arksey and O'Malley 2005) and refined for clinical practice in the mid-2010s (Peters et al. 2015).

Instead of ES's usual goal of hypothesis-testing (Tricco et al. 2016), scoping reviews use ES aggregation methods to scope what literature exists on a subject. By completing a scoping review, researchers might gain a meta-understanding of their query—a better sense of the type of publications published on a subject, when a topic was studied, or other aspects of the research landscape itself. In particular, scoping reviews can be "useful tools for evidence reconnaissance [that] can be used to provide a broad overview of a topic. For instance, a scoping review that seeks to develop a 'concept map' may aim to explore how, by whom, and for what purpose *a particular term* is used in a given field" (Peters et al. 2020, emphasis added).

I applied scoping review methodology to collect and map subject vocabulary collocated with the term *food studies* across five large bibliographic databases chosen for size, relevance, and metadata standards. I searched ProQuest Central, EBSCO Discovery Service, Web of Science, PubMed, and PubAg. In each, I searched the phrase "food studies," selected the peer-review filters (where possible), and extracted the results. Pooled together and de-duplicated, I had an exhaustive set of 5,666 articles with the phrase "food studies" somewhere in their metadata. However, I found that there were many false positives. These mainly originated from circumstances of coincidental phrasing from a scholar describing plural dietary investigations. (For example, W. D. Rundle's [1982] article "A Case for Esophageal Analysis in Shorebird Food Studies" synthesizes multiple reports about the eating habits of waterfowl; it is not an article on avian gastronomy or systems.) To determine true or false positives, I manually checked each of the 5,666 records. Ultimately, after sifting through the results, I validated that 3,365 articles had the moniker "food studies" somewhere in their metadata. (This means that in all journal literature, the phrase "food studies" relates to the field only about 59.39 percent of the time.) The corpus of positive results is henceforth referred to as the Food Studies Corpus (FSC) (Malin 2020).

Although one could (and I plan to in the future) study the FSC's thousands of articles' full-texts, for this project these were not the data I analyzed. Instead I studied their metadata records. Like many databases, each of the 3,365 records in the FCS contains a subject keyword section describing the article's content. I focused on studying these subject keywords. By enumerating the usage of these subject keywords and their relative cooccurrences, we may better understand how they exist across academic databases. Generally, disciplinary keyword analysis is used to identify significant aspects of a well-trod field in a predetermined domain (Chen and Xiao 2014). However, I employed these bibliometric techniques in the opposite direction. In this case, subject keyword frequency gave a stipulative description of the field: an exhaustive list of enumerated words (and thus the concepts they represent) and the amount each is used relative to others. However, because keyword frequency results rely on counting exact textual strings, I first had to cluster and merge these subject keywords in a process called crosswalking (Sundar et al. 2008). To do so, I used five algorithmic methods available in data cleaning software (OpenRefine) and manually validated every merge. From this process, I found that approximately 26 percent of the original 11,678 subject keywords were duplicates, with only slight grammatical variations. This left 8,632 unique subject keywords—a list of concepts that (in theory, exhaustively) described the entire field's article research content.

To understand each subject keyword's preponderance and relationships I mapped them with Visualization of Similarity Viewer (VOS-Viewer). The complete and interactive map is available at online (Malin 2023). VOSViewer, released by Netherlands-based developers Nees Jan van Eck and Ludo Waltman in 2009, "aims to provide a low-dimensional visualization in which objects are located in such a way that the distance between any pair of objects reflects their similarity as accurately as possible" (Van Eck and Waltman 2007, 305). The software's keyword co-word function creates a network "based on the co-occurrence of pairs of words, [and therefore] co-word analysis seeks to extract the themes of science and detect the linkages among these themes directly from the subject content of texts." (Sedighi 2016, 53). VOSViewer's co-word method is an excellent tool to "predict the relationship between research fronts of a discipline and related literature" (Qiu et al. 2017, 329).

In my "food studies" map, nodes are subject keywords, and the distance and orientation among nodes are based on algorithmically calculated relevance scores. The lines in the visualization show the connection of at least two article records that share a subject keyword. As is explained by Bornmann, Haunschild, and Hug (2018), "The distance between two subject [keywords or] headings (two nodes) is approximately inversely proportional to the similarity (relatedness in terms co-occurrence) of the keywords. Hence, subject keywords with a higher co-occurrence rate tend to be found closer to each other" (430).

With this map, scholars can make some interesting meta-observations. For example, although the terms *nutrition* and *diet* are colloquially synonymous, the map shows clearly that they have vastly different meanings in research. *Nutrition* skews to the map's center, alluding to its broader use than *diet*, which is used a similar amount but cleanly sits in the dietetics cluster. This shows scientifically a difference between these two terms that scholars previously could intuit only after years of practice; that, for example, a researcher studying macronutrient intake, health determinants, disease comorbidities, and other scientific attributes of consumption should use the term *diet*, but any scholar looking for cultural, historical, political, or other social aspects of consumption uses the term *nutrition* instead. This map's complexity and size, therefore, make these and other subject keyword relationships a new and meaningful way to understand the field.

Conclusion

No matter the discipline, there is always some linguistic disconnect between the words scholars choose to write with and the words researchers decide to search for. Comfort with navigating a field's particular subject keywords is usually a signifier of academic mastery and experience. This is not true for food studies, however. As a new and multidisciplinary field, food studies' nascence precludes any requisite cannon of materials or a strict oeuvre of methodology. Its diverse objectives and perspectives enable researchers to work among numerous lineages of academic thought. Unfortunately, the food studies community has not communicated the ramifications of its diffuse scholarly landscape well, resulting in perceived deviance. This ontological flexibility correlates to similar real-life issues, beyond those in bibliographic research. For example, Bellows and colleagues (2018) showed routine difficulties in tenure and promotion processes. The field's diffuse scholarly landscape may have had a hand in that. For example, what must a promotion panel think when they cannot find their new food-focused sociology fellow's articles in SocINDEX? Would they trust the scrutiny of a conference paper refereed by a rag-tag assortment of PhD fields as much as they trust the rigor of their sociology peers?

While food studies leaders work to fix these optics, the community should discuss more the nature and qualities of its own research landscape. It is up to scholars to choose how to marshal cohesion out of disorder and how much they are willing to communicate in nonstandard dialects. In the meantime, I hope librarians begin to support liminal academic spaces with intent, rather than allowing them to slip between subject cracks. By removing the yoke of subject specificity and focusing on the particular needs of cross-disciplines themselves, librarians may begin to help. In doing so librarians may begin to cook for the chefs in the scholarly kitchen and help sustain food scholars for years to come.

REFERENCES

Arksey, Hilary, and Lisa O'Malley. 2005. "Scoping Studies: Towards a Methodological Framework." *International Journal of Social Research Methodology* 8, no. 1 (February): 19–32. https://doi.org/10.1080/1364557032000119616.

Astroff, Roberta. 2012. "The Structuring Work of Disciplines." In *Interdisciplinarity and Academic Libraries*, edited by Daniel C Mack and Craig Gibson, 5–16. ACRL Publications in Librarianship 66. Chicago: Association of College and Research Libraries.

Bates, Marcia J. 1996. "Learning about the Information Seeking of Interdisciplinary Scholars and Students." *Library Trends* 45, no. 2 (Fall): 155–64.

Belasco, Warren James. 2008. *Food: The Key Concepts*. Oxford: Berg.

Bellows, Anne, Rick Welsh, Maize Ludden, and Briana Alfaro. 2018. "Promotion and Tenure, Journals, and Impact Factor in the Field of Food Studies: Results from May 2017 Qualtrics Survey." Association for the Study of Food and Society. Food-culture.org.

Bornmann, Lutz, Robin Haunschild, and Sven E. Hug. 2018. "Visualizing the Context of Citations Referencing Papers Published by Eugene Garfield: A New Type of Keyword Co-Occurrence Analysis." *Scientometrics* 114, no. 2 (December): 427–37. https://doi.org/10.1007/s11192-017-2591-8.

Chen, Guo, and Lu Xiao. 2016. "Selecting Publication Keywords for Domain Analysis in Bibliometrics: A Comparison of Three Methods." *Journal of Informetrics* 10, no. 1 (February): 212–23. https://doi.org/10.1016/j.joi.2016.01.006.

Choi, Bernard C. K., and Anita W. P. Pak. 2006. "Multidisciplinarity, Interdisciplinarity and Transdisciplinarity in Health Research, Services, Education and Policy: 1. Definitions, Objectives, and Evidence of Effectiveness." *Clinical and Investigative Medicine* 29, no. 6 (December): 351–64.

Cochrane, Archibald Leman. 2004. *Effectiveness and Efficiency: Random Reflections on Health Services*. The Rock Carling Fellowship 1971. London: Royal Society of Medicine Press.

Duran, Nancy, and Karen MacDonald. 2006. "Information Sources for Food Studies Research." *Food, Culture & Society* 9 (2): 233–43. https://doi.org/10.2752/1552 80106778606080.

Fuller, Steve. 2013. "Deviant Interdisciplinarity as Philosophical Practice: Prolegomena to Deep Intellectual History." *Synthese* 190, no. 11 (October): 1899–1916. https://doi .org/10.1007/s11229-012-0208-6.

Gullbekk, Eystein, Idunn Bøyum, and Katriina Byström. 2015. "Interdisciplinarity and Information Literacy: Librarians' Competencies in Emerging Settings of Higher Education." *Proceedings of the Association for Information Science and Technology* 52 (1): 1–4. https://doi.org/10.1002/pra2.2015.145052010079.

Hagell, A. and Bourke Dowling, S. 1999. "Scoping Review of Literature on the Health and Care of Mentally Disordered Offenders." *CRD Report* 16. York: NHS Centre for Reviews and Dissemination, University of York. https://www.york.ac.uk.

Hamada, Shingo, Richard Wilk, Amanda Logan, Sara Minard, and Amy Trubek. 2015. "The Future of Food Studies." *Food, Culture & Society* 18, no. 1 (April): 167–86. https://doi.org/10.2752/175174415X14101814953846.

Heldke, Lisa. 2006. "The Unexamined Meal Is Not Worth Eating: Or, Why and How Philosophers (Might/Could/Do) Study Food." *Food, Culture & Society* 9, no. 2 (April): 201–19. https://doi.org/10.2752/155280106778606035.

Hjørland, Birger. 2005. "Domain Analysis: A Socio-Cognitive Orientation for Information Science Research." *Bulletin of the American Society for Information Science and Technology* 30, no. 3 (January): 17–21. https://doi.org/10.1002/bult.312.

———. 2009. "Concept Theory." *Journal of the American Society for Information Science and Technology* 60, no. 8 (April): 1519–36. https://doi.org/10.1002/asi.21082.

———. 2011. "The Importance of Theories of Knowledge: Indexing and Information Retrieval as an Example." *Journal of the American Society for Information Science and Technology* 62, no. 1 (November): 72–77. https://doi.org/10.1002/asi.21451.

Huutoniemi, Katri, Julie Thompson Klein, Henrik Bruun, and Janne Hukkinen. 2010. "Analyzing Interdisciplinarity: Typology and Indicators." *Research Policy* 39, no. 1 (February): 79–88. https://doi.org/10.1016/j.respol.2009.09.011.

Klein, Julie T. 2015. "Interdisciplinarity and Collaboration." In *Ethics, Science, Technology, and Engineering: A Global Resource*, 2nd ed., edited by J. Britt Holbrook and Carl Mitcham, 576–78. Farmington Hills, MI: Gale, Cengage Learning/Macmillan Reference USA.

Klein, Julie T., and Carl Mitcham. 2010. "A Taxonomy of Interdisciplinarity." In *The Oxford Handbook of Interdisciplinarity*, edited by Robert Frodeman, 15–30. New York: Oxford University Press.

Korr, Jeremy L., and Christine Broussard. 2004. "Challenges in the Interdisciplinary Teaching of Food and Foodways." *Food, Culture & Society* 7, no. 2 (April): 147–59. https://doi.org/10.2752/155280104786577941.

Larivière, Vincent, Stefanie Haustein, and Philippe Mongeon. 2015. "The Oligopoly of Academic Publishers in the Digital Era." *PLOS ONE* 10, no. 6 (June). https://doi.org/10.1371/journal.pone.0127502.

Malin, James E. 2020. "The 'Food Studies' Corpus." Open Science Framework. https://doi.org/10.17605/OSF.IO/DV57F.

———. 2023. "The 'Food Studies' Corpus Map." VOSViewer Online. https://tinyurl.com/28r8thd4.

Nestle, Marion, and W. Alex McIntosh. 2010. "Writing the Food Studies Movement." *Food, Culture & Society* 13, no. 2 (April): 159–79. https://doi.org/10.2752/175174410X12633934462999.

Olson, Hope A. 2008. "How We Construct Subjects: A Feminist Analysis." *Library Trends* 56, no. 2 (Fall): 509–41. https://doi.org/10.1353/lib.2008.0007.

Peters, Micah D. J., Christina M. Godfrey, Hanan Khalil, Patricia McInerney, Deborah Parker, and Cassia Baldini Soares. 2015. "Guidance for Conducting Systematic Scoping Reviews:" *International Journal of Evidence-Based Healthcare* 13, no. 3 (September): 141–46. https://doi.org/10.1097/XEB.0000000000000050.

Peters, Micah, Christina Godfrey, Patricia McInerney, Zachary Munn, Andrea Tricco, and Hanan Khalil. 2020. "Scoping Reviews (2020 version)." In *The Joanna Briggs Institute Manual for Evidence Synthesis*, edited by Edoardo Aromataris and Zachary Munn. South Australia: Joanna Briggs Institute. https://doi.org/10.46658/JBIMES-20-12.

Qiu, Junping, Rongying Zhao, Siluo Yang, and Ke Dong. 2017. *Informetrics*. Singapore: Springer Singapore. https://doi.org/10.1007/978-981-10-4032-0.

Rundle, W. Dean. 1982. "A Case for Esophageal Analysis in Shorebird Food Studies." *Journal of Field Ornithology* 53, no. 3 (Summer): 249–57.

Sedighi, Mehri. 2016. "Application of Word Co-Occurrence Analysis Method in Mapping of the Scientific Fields (Case Study: The Field of Informetrics)." *Library Review* 65. no. 1/2 (February): 52–64. https://doi.org/10.1108/LR-07-2015-0075.

Sundar, Vidyalakshmi, Marcia E. Daumen, Daniel J. Conley, and John H. Stone. 2008. "The Use of ICF Codes for Information Retrieval in Rehabilitation Research: An Empirical Study." *Disability and Rehabilitation* 30 (12–13): 955–62. https://doi.org/10.1080/09638280701800285.

Tricco, Andrea C., Erin Lillie, Wasifa Zarin, Kelly O'Brien, Heather Colquhoun, Monika Kastner, Danielle Levac, et al. 2016. "A Scoping Review on the Conduct and Reporting of Scoping Reviews." *BMC Medical Research Methodology* 16 (1): 15. https://doi.org/10.1186/s12874-016-0116-4.

Van Eck, Nees Jan, and Ludo Waltman. 2007. "VOS: A New Method for Visualizing Similarities Between Objects." In *Advances in Data Analysis*, edited by Reinhold Decker and Hans-J. Lenz, 299–306. Berlin: Springer. https://doi.org/10.1007/978-3-540-70981-7_34.

13

Action Research and Social Engagement

Food Studies in Practice

AMY BENTLEY, JENNIFER BERG, CAROLYN DIMITRI, MARION NESTLE, FABIO PARASECOLI, KRISHNENDU RAY

As mentioned in the introduction and demonstrated throughout the chapters of this volume, NYU food studies is a product of its location (New York City, New York University, a professionally oriented school within NYU, and a department shared with a nutrition program) as well as its methodologically and disciplinarily diverse faculty. The program is also very much part of the development of food studies as a field, contributing to its evolving dialogue with food cultures and food systems around the world and its growing desire to address their most urgent issues. Moreover, NYU food studies is shaped by its orientation to its students, the majority of whom are pursuing master's degrees with an eye toward employment in the private or public sectors (as opposed to academia). To that end, as faculty, our research and fieldwork tend to lean toward scholarship with an interdisciplinary, applied bent.

This is partly the result of the abovementioned physical realities and pragmatic considerations. We are in a professional school that trains professionals for "real-world" jobs, for example, and our course content—assignments and projects—is designed with an eye toward this goal. Further, we believe in the necessity of teaching the subject of food from an interdisciplinary perspective. There is no other way that approaches the topic thoroughly and provides knowledge and experience that can help solve real world problems. Finally, our scholarship, similar to our teaching, is at the intersection of application and theory.

Our scholarship and fieldwork tend to be located within this intersection not only because we find the problems there important, but because the theoretical perspectives many of us find compelling push us in this direction. These often focus around issues of power and agency: Can mere humans, for example, effect change in the face of huge, seemingly insurmountable institutions of power and privilege? Instead of admitting defeat by "wicked" problems in the food system, how can we take back ownership and agency—how can we make a difference? Thus, the work of French culture theorist Michel de Certeau is compelling. His book *The Practice of Everyday Life* finds human agency in small everyday tasks such as walking, talking, reading, and cooking, "tactics" that counter the power of institutions, entities, and persons with power and wealth (1984). The mundane task of cooking, tiny as it is, may then contribute to countering large food corporations' attempts to dominate food choices, habits, and health. Similarly relevant and compelling is the work of British sociologist Alan Warde and his notion of *practice theory* (2014, 2016). Meaning, instead of residing in things or ideas, is located in practices and actions. Culture is something humans "do," which again points to human action and agency as key. These theoretical underpinnings provide ballast for scholarship that is focused on community engagement, is interdisciplinary in nature, and addresses real-world problems. In a broader political and cultural sense, there is a premium on maintaining this perspective. This optimistic perspective may be labeled naive by some, but the current global political climate, for example with its growing fascist impulses, requires that humans retain some sense of agency to counter the ominous institutional powers and pressures. For this reason, methodologies such participatory action research, codesign, public humanities, and other forms of embedded and practice-based and community-engaged scholarship are becoming increasingly relevant in a field that deals with urgent issues that cannot be addressed by academics only (Chevalier and Buckles 2019; Gordon Da Cruz 2018; Manzini 2015).

Recounted in first person, NYU food studies faculty members explain here how they have translated food studies into practice, and in doing so the following themes emerge: advocacy, professional expertise and assistance, experiential education, and public programming and knowledge creation. Although we thought it was important to hear the individual voices of those involved, these experiences are examples of the increasingly engaged work and research that is emerging in food studies as a field, shaping its present while pointing to the future.

Advocacy: Marion Nestle and Krishnendu Ray describe their work as advocates for public policy and social justice, highlighting Nestle's work on behalf of the Mexico soda tax initiative and Ray's work with New York City's Street Vendor Project.

Professional Expertise Sharing: Carolyn Dimitri and Fabio Parasecoli discuss their collaborations with others with the goal of improving food systems nationally and globally. Dimitri describes her involvement in NGOs that seek to reduce social/environmental costs of conventional agriculture, and Parasecoli, with colleagues in Poland, establishes collaborative partnerships that strengthen commitments to food in academic and public settings.

Experiential Education: Jennifer Berg and Amy Bentley describe their efforts to enhance the classroom experience. Berg discusses food studies travel courses that take students deep into the NYC outer boroughs as well as globally, and Bentley and Berg describe the NYU Urban Farm Lab experiential hands-on learning lab for teaching and research.

Public Programming and Knowledge Creation: Amy Bentley discusses two collaborative public-facing entities, the Experimental Cuisine Collective and the Food and COVID-19 NYC Digital Archive and Collection, designed not only to appeal to the general public but to involve them in knowledge making.

Advocacy

Marion Nestle

I want my applied work in food politics to inspire students and anyone else it reaches to become advocates for healthier and more sustainable food systems. My purpose in writing articles and books, teaching, giving public lectures, and talking to media reporters is to explain how almost everything about food involves politics and how necessary it is to engage in politics if we want to improve dietary health and planetary sustainability.

That is why I teach food advocacy. The basis of successful advocacy is well established. Advocates must define a clear goal and identify precisely what they want to achieve or change. They must do their homework and provide data and documentation for the need for that change. They must locate a specific target of their campaign—the person or institution with the power to make the desired change. They must convince as many people and groups as possible to join them in their cause. Building community is the key to successful advocacy; campaigns require a broad base of public support. Working closely with allies, advocates must develop strategies to convince their target to act, and then they must implement those strategies. If their campaign fails, they need to analyze why and start over. Standard advocacy methods are entirely analogous to those taught in program planning and policy development courses offered by schools of public health and public policy. To the extent that advocates adhere to theoretical methods—especially those that involve community support—their campaigns are likely to succeed.

I do not have the temperament to be an on-the-ground community organizer. Instead, I see my role as developing the research basis for food advocacy, as I did in my book *Soda Politics: Taking on Big Food (and Winning)*. I intended this book as an advocacy manual for campaigns to reduce consumption of sugar-sweetened beverages by taxing them, removing them from schools, stopping companies from marketing them to children, and placing warning labels on soda cans and bottles. I wrote my book with Kerry Trueman, *Let's Ask Marion*, to convince students and readers that engaging in politics is essential for creating more democratic and more equitable food systems, those that will prevent hunger, promote public health, and prevent environmental damage. I have been accused of writing polemics and am guilty as charged, but I document what I write as carefully as I can, and in great detail.

In recent years, I have presented the results of my research to advocates for food and nutrition policy in Australia, for soda taxes in Mexico, for warning labels on ultra-processed foods in Chile, and for curbing corporate involvement in nutrition policy in China, Brazil, and Israel, to pick a few examples. Throughout the world, food advocates face similar barriers: weak government support, a largely disengaged civil society, strong and well-organized food industry opposition, and lack of financial resources.

Despite these challenges, advocacy groups have found ways to gain enough support to make real progress on food issues through sound research, clear identification of goals and targets, and close attention to building community coalitions. These skills necessarily draw on lessons learned from sociology, anthropology, political science, economics, and public health science.

Another example: I used a Fulbright Specialist Fellowship developed in collaboration with Mexico's Instituto Nacional de Salud Pública (National Institute of Public Health) to collaborate with the institute's team working on chronic disease prevention. These researchers and their civil society partners, most notably El Poder del Consumidor (consumer power) and its coalition of advocacy groups, La Alianza por la Salud Alimentaria (nutritional health alliance), had succeeded in getting the Mexican government to tax sugar-sweetened beverages and were evaluating its effects and pressing for improvements in the policy. The alliance, working with the Public Health Institute, had accomplished this by drawing on the full range of interdisciplinary skills required for public health planning, implementation, and evaluation: research, target setting, coalition building, strategic planning, media work, and resource acquisition. The strength of these skills—and their potential for success—was so apparent that the Bloomberg Foundation volunteered to fund the work of these groups and did, generously. My role was to give lectures on the broader public health and international context of the Mexican soda tax initiatives and to publicly provide international support for the work of this advocacy alliance. If my work can contribute to such efforts, I consider it entirely worth the time and effort I put into it.

Krishnendu Ray

One of my objectives has been to work directly with groups and organizations fighting for social justice for workers of color. I have sought that by diffusing my research with the goal of strengthening democracy from below. The successful passage of Bill 1116B by the NYC Council on January 28, 2021, marked an important step toward that goal. We worked for a decade on that project, fund-raising, lobbying city and state government, launching social media campaigns, and pounding the pavement to organize street vendors, most of whom are people of color, often refugees and undocumented immigrants (Street Vendor Project n.d.). There are currently 3,900 vending permits in New York City, most of which are traded on the black market at about $20,000 per permit. Vendors must buy those permits or risk operating on the streets without the requisite documentation, which can lead to hefty fines, confiscation of equipment, and/or arrests. The bill passed by the City Council seeks to reform these elements.

The bill will make more permits available and affordable and create a new enforcement agency that will lead to less criminal liability, particularly for immigrants, who constitute most of New York City's street food vendors. Over the next ten years, the new bill will add four thousand more permits and will retire old tradable permits. I was one of the seven-member advisory board and strategic planning leadership of the Street Vendor Project on this initiative to pass the new law. Over the last decade, I have worked to provide testimony to the New York City Council and the mayor, undertaking research on vendor livelihoods, hosting fundraising activities, generating support in the public domain, and participating in membership drives. In 2021, we delivered $2,305,000 in financial relief to city street vendors, helping 2,333 vendors, in particular 1,100 non-citizen vendors with the Excluded Workers Fund, and we assisted 450 vendors with legal aid.

It is the advocacy work in New York City that shaped my next research project on street vendors. A global consortium of scholars built a website to collaborate and learn from each other while trying to develop a theory that could account for street vending in the Global North and the Global South. The work led to a special issue of the journal *Food, Culture & Society* in which teams reported their findings (Allison, Ray, and Rohel 2021). Our team was already interviewing street vendors in India and working with WIEGO (Women in the Informal Economy: Globalizing and Organizing), one of the earliest working-class feminist organizations in the Global South, when COVID-19 hit. Vendors were so acutely affected that we decided to re-deploy our resources to grasp the ongoing challenges of vendor lives and provide aid where possible. We worked on fundraising, distributing provisions, and putting pressure on the national, regional, and local governments to provide free transportation back home, housing subsidies, and ration cards.

In India, it is estimated that anywhere between four to ten million people make their living on the streets, selling produce in markets and neighborhoods and cooked food at bus stands, train stations, traffic roundabouts, parks, and on sidewalks. In New Delhi alone it is estimated that there are around three hundred thousand street vendors (about half of them migrants). Once India commenced a stringent lockdown on March 24, 2020, with no planning, millions of poor workers had a mere four-hour's notice to get back to their homes of origin or survive in their migrant abodes in the megacities. What was needed was much better information at the ground level and greater investment in the infrastructure to support the lives of the poor—the focus of our efforts with WIEGO and Janpahal, another organization.

This advocacy work is shaping my next book, *The Death of the Street Vendor*, which will investigate the role played by the informal sector in maintaining the livelihoods and markets necessary for the survival of the poor in the Global South. Over the last fifty years, there has been a rich and burgeoning literature on *urban informality*. Informality is by definition what has *not* been captured by large corporate capital or by the state, things that are neither particularly profitable nor necessary to accumulate substantial power. It is fundamentally a small-scale bazaar commercialism that preceded capitalism, exceeds its grasp today, and will in all probability survive it.

For over the last five hundred years, capitalism has been the dominant historical relationship between large states, emerging in the Mediterranean and Atlantic worlds and then spreading elsewhere (Banaji 2020; Braudel 1984). In *Rethinking Capitalist Development* (2014), the Indian economist Kalyan Sanyal brings that analysis up to the contemporary moment in a highly celebrated critique that the bazaar economy of petty transactions is the domain of need rather than capital accumulation. It is not a transitional stage to some better form of capitalism but permanently in place, contrary to the claims of Marxist theorists or anti-Marxist liberal developmentalists. The system is built to keep millions of people outside the domain of the main channels of capital accumulation. Yet it is a system forced on the state in the wake of the victory of anticolonial nationalism and popular sovereignty (RoyChowdhury 2021). That is the basis of the current state of the vendor economy which feeds most people in the Global South. My advocacy work is leading back into my professional research.

Professional Expertise Sharing

Carolyn Dimitri

My research and outreach activities reflect my beliefs about the food system, that the process of producing, distributing, and consuming food creates environmental and social costs external to the food's production.

Thus, from a social welfare perspective, the farms and firms that constitute the food system produce too much environmental degradation and excessively high human costs. In addition to writing and thinking about the external costs, I provide service to society by participating in groups that seek to ameliorate these costs. I am an applied economist and have a strong belief in markets. However, I recognize that the private sector's needs will never be completely aligned with public interest, particularly if it means that profits will be reduced. Thus, as part of this work, I discuss the importance of recognizing social and environmental costs, which includes thinking about how farmers, firms, and consumers will respond to changes in prices or other incentives.

Three areas of volunteer service have been in the form of board participation: the executive board of the Organic Farming Research Foundation, the now defunct Organic and Regenerative Agriculture Advisory Council to General Mills, and the federal advisory committee to the USDA's National Organic Program (NOP), the National Organic Standards Board (NOSB). The missions of these three groups—representing the nonprofit sector, the private sector, and the federal government—coalesce around a common theme of supporting organic agriculture, a farming system where farmers develop agricultural production in harmony with the agroecosystem, minimizing damage to soil, biodiversity, and water bodies, and reducing emission of greenhouse gasses.

In practice, however, organic agriculture faces numerous hurdles. Federal support of organic farming is significantly smaller than federal support of conventional agriculture, meaning that many organic farmers do not receive funding for participating in conservation programs; crop insurance is more difficult to purchase, and organic farmers may be excluded from disaster payment programs. The lack of federal support has historically meant that funding is less available for research on organic farming and marketing practices. The Organic Farming Research Foundation has attempted to fill in the lack of research funding by providing small grants to allow researchers and farmers to conduct early research on matters important to the organic sector. In 2021, the research funding program specifically targeted early career researchers along with Black, Indigenous, and people of color researchers to provide funding for projects led by scientists and scholars who tend to be underserved in the federal research realm.

The organic food system, like the overall food system, operates in a market, and thus private led initiatives can be an important mechanism for change. The General Mills Organic and Regenerative Advisory Council consisted of farmers, researchers, and General Mills employees to brainstorm ways that the company could increase the supply of organic products. While doing so was clearly in alignment with their goals of building demand for their packaged food products with younger households (twenty-five to forty-five years of age), the entire group was committed to important social goals: preserving farmland for future production, supporting farm income, and mitigating climate change through enhanced agricultural practices.

When the Organic Foods Production Act was passed in the 1990 Farm Bill, the authors were keenly aware of the potential for greenwashing and eroding the organic standards. Undoubtedly, as the organic industry grew, with increased participation of large multinational food companies, the pressure to relax the organic standards would be fierce. Thus, the act created a volunteer advisory committee, the National Organic Standards Board (NOSB), with representatives from all parts of the organic community: consumers, the environment, organic farmers, organic certifiers, retailers, and a scientist with expertise in toxicology, ecology, or biochemistry. The board members are appointed for staggered five-year terms. At the time of this writing, as an NOSB board member, I currently represent the interests of consumers. The NOSB meets publicly and is prohibited from meeting privately as an entire board, with the hope that the process of discussing policies and allowable ingredients is transparent.

The political pressure on the board can be aptly described through the case of carrageenan, a seaweed-derived additive widely used as a thickener in non-dairy milks. The product came up for sunset review, which happens every five years, in 2016, when the NOSB voted to delist the product, as the board felt the additive did not meet the standards for ingredients allowed in organic processed products. The NOP, however, determined that carrageenan was "essential" to organic production and disregarded the NOSB's recommendation to delist. Despite the NOP's claim that the product was essential, many food manufacturers were able to reformulate their products to use other products. Fast-forward five years, when carrageenan was reviewed again, as required by law. This time, however, the NOSB voted 9–5 to delist, which missed the threshold for delisting by one vote. The change in the vote was largely the result of several new members who voted in the interest of corporate needs rather than consumer demands or respecting the unanimous vote of the 2016 board. The composition of the board clearly matters, and the organic community has often pointed to the fact that some of the seats are awarded to individuals with strong corporate ties rather than a commitment to improving planetary health through organic farming.

My volunteer work on boards supports my teaching and research and provides me with some interesting fodder to share with my students. The work is frustrating, though, as I believe some (particularly those on the NOSB) put the needs of their corporations over society. Pressure on the private sector in the form of consumer demand and government regulation is critical to preserving the health of the ecosystem, which includes supporting healthy levels of biodiversity and minimizing environmental degradation. The food system needs to be both resilient and sustainable—as a system. In my view, organic farming systems are a key part of helping the food system achieve resiliency and sustainability and to allowing the agroecosystem to support future generations by producing healthy and nourishing food. That vision is what inspires me to contribute my time and expertise to our future.

Fabio Parasecoli

An important aspect of being part of a university with global outreach is establishing collaborations with institutions and scholars in other countries. These encounters force us to rethink the way we work, our methodologies, and our theoretical background, as everything suddenly appears much more relative and we realize that there are diverse and legitimate points of views and customs that are radically different from ours. Although this would seem evident, when we face these differences in the practicalities of research, we acknowledge that they are deeply connected to power imbalances that are themselves tied not only to academic systems but also to larger geopolitical dynamics. I will use as an example the research project, launched with funding from the Narodowe Centrum Nauki (National Science Centre) of Poland, on which I worked between 2018 and 2022. The investigation explored the ongoing revaluation of Polish food in terms of space through the rearticulation of the categories of local, regional, and national, and time through discourses around history and tradition.

As I write these paragraphs, the research is being developed into a book, in collaboration with Mateusz Halawa, an anthropologist and ethnographer from the Institute of Philosophy and Sociology at the Polish Academy of Sciences, and Agata Bachórz, a sociologist from the University of Gdańsk. In fact, the reflections that follow are the result of our shared conversations, as coauthors. The power relations between the societies and the academic worlds from which we come constitute the background of our collaboration; a center-periphery frame is an accurate conceptualization of this relationship. Because of this, there are significant differences between our situations, which affect our positionality in and outside of academia and the methods and the practices we embrace (Bachórz and Parasecoli 2020).

Mateusz and Agata, although Polish, are in some ways outsiders to the local food industry; although an outsider to Poland, I am well known among Polish tastemakers as a food scholar and a journalist. The international prestige of NYU, my global experience, and my Italian ethnicity create an expectation of culinary competence, making access to the industry easy but complicating the relationship with our interlocutors, who are constantly pulling me into their ranks for visibility, social currency, and advice.

They see a confirmation of the value of Polish food in my interest in it and in my engagement with them. I have also been invited to be a judge in culinary contests for specialties I was not previously familiar with, from *pierogi* to *nalewki* (infusion liquors) and *czernina* (duck blood soup) precisely because of my position as a foreigner with different taste categories. My participation was actually welcome to give more gravitas, status, and visibility to the contests and their participants.

When food professionals launched the idea of a Twaróg Day as a way to celebrate a simple but ubiquitous traditional (and often handmade) fresh cheese, I was invited to be one of the signatories of the document, which points to how I am now considered not only an observer but actually a participant in the changes taking place in the Polish foodscape (the declaration expressed both the respect for existing practice and the desire to elevate the product to better fit higher standards of quality and taste). These dynamics prompt us to ask questions about the limits of

intervention into the researched reality as well as the source of this am-
biguous and not entirely equal relation between the researcher and the
field. In line with a postcolonial pattern, recognition still comes from
outside.

Mateusz's and Agata's roles and interventions in the research are more
difficult to describe because they are not so visible in the food industry;
there are not many ethnographic facts to recall as in my case. They had
fewer previous experiences of engagement with food-related activities in
non-academic roles. What is particularly interesting, their role is rarely
linked to the evaluation of food as such in terms of taste, quality, or authenticity. They are usually well received by our interlocutors, but their
presence in the field is not particularly sought after and often has to
do with the limited time of their potential interviewees. Perhaps it is to
some extent a delusion of "transparency," but it can be assumed that the
motivations of their interlocutors are less instrumental and the relations
turn out to be less hierarchical. In general they have not felt they had any
debt to (symbolically) pay back, which is good for a critical approach.

Our own experience highlights many advantages in having different backgrounds, points of views, and even methodological approaches
among co-researchers, as long as we maintain a self-reflective attitude
and we are not afraid of discussing our own roles and our own entangle-
ments with power structures. While trying not to sound paternalistic
and avoiding any unilinear evolutionary framework when juxtaposing
the two academias in which we operate (Poland and the United States)
and the transition of food research into food studies, we use our own
experiences as "lessons learned" in order to underscore the fact that it is
impossible to disconnect the politics of food from the politics of doing
food research in terms of involvement with power structures, hierarchies, and hegemonic dynamics, both in the public sphere and within
academia itself.

Experiential Education

Jennifer Berg

In 2007, as New York City was rebounding from 9/11, with immigration patterns in flux, I developed the course Field Trips in Food:
Immigrant New York City as a way for graduate students to understand

and explore New York's immigrant-dominated neighborhoods. Given the richness of the material, deciding which communities and themes to focus on proved a challenge. Options included nostalgic spaces (the Lower East Side), historically significant neighborhoods (Little Italy), emerging immigrant groups (Egyptians in Queens), tourist draws (Manhattan's Chinatown), and population surges (Dominican Washington Heights). Ultimately, I structured the course around six themes: immigration and acculturation, the performance and mythology of cultural identity, redefining marginalized groups through racial or linguistic similarities, religion as unifier and barrier, economic stratification, and the effects of global crisis. The course has proved a great success and is offered each year.

In advance of each weekly tour, students explore an array of related materials including census reports, memoirs, historical accounts, newspaper articles, maps, and video clips. Traversing the boroughs, we travel together by subway discussing the week's literature and themes. Markets, bakeries, parks, architecture, public schools, grocery stores, street vendors, residential options, street-level stores, and religious centers all contribute to engaging with and understanding a community's historical and cultural landscape. For example, for the week entitled Global South in Queens we zigzag across Elmhurst, Corona, and Jackson Heights taking in the sounds, aromas, and tastes of a community. The neighborhood, originally developed as a restricted, lily-white enclave, has become one of the most linguistically, ethnically, racially, and economically diverse areas in the United States. We trace the demographic evolution, from its white Christian origin to mid-century influx of Puerto Rican migrants, to a late-twentieth-century wave of South American immigration (Columbian, Ecuadorean, Guatemalan, Salvadorean, Peruvian, and Uruguayan), to the most recent immigration from central Mexico. Through each of these waves, we see how broader narratives and overarching generalizations define and often distort the community.

For their final research projects, students create interactive historical maps that highlight the role that food plays in defining a neighborhood throughout decades of demographic change. Projects focus on, for example, well-established groups (Koreans in Midtown Manhattan), communities in demographic decline (Italians on Arthur Avenue in the Bronx), or communities that wax and wane in response to global economic swings (Greeks in Astoria, Queens). Other projects explore emerging communities (Sri Lankan in Staten Island), lost communities (Norwegians in south Brooklyn), and those with distinct historical nostalgia (Germans in Yorkville). The projects do not remain static. Given New York City's ongoing demographic diversification and subsequent neighborhood changes, students often update their projects after graduation.

In addition to the local field trips course, our commitment to experiential interdisciplinary education extends beyond Greenwich Village and New York City. Each year, NYU food studies offers a handful of graduate immersive short-term study abroad options (we also offer on occasion a more limited number of specialized courses for undergraduate honors students). Many courses have been located at one of the fourteen NYU global campuses (Italy, France, Berlin, Prague, Shanghai, and Washington, DC), while others are separate endeavors at locations chosen for significant geographical anomalies (India, New Orleans, Puerto Rico, Ireland). Over the course of several weeks, a food studies faculty member steers twelve to sixteen students through farms, markets, religious sites, museums, food production facilities, wineries, breweries, guided tastings, tours, and guest lectures. In the past few years, students have explored the resurgence of Irish independence and identity via food, food in socialist and post-socialist economies in Berlin and Prague, the performance of modern French identity in Paris, the Mediterranean diet in Italy, capitalism and industrialization in Shanghai, the Columbian exchange in Mexico, global capitalism and settler colonialism via sugar in Puerto Rico, organic food policy in Washington, DC, and social hierarchy in India.

NYU Urban Farm Lab
Amy Bentley and Jennifer Berg

The NYU Urban Farm Lab is a small plot of land facing six lanes of Manhattan traffic with a year-round thriving program in urban agriculture. Here, NYU graduate and undergraduate students participate in the Urban Agriculture class (currently taught by urban farm manager Melissa Metrick) and get hands-on training and experience in the practice of organic agricultural techniques. In addition, the NYU Urban Farm Lab also serves social and cultural functions by bringing communities (local nursery school, residents, student groups, researchers and others) together through soil preparation, seed germination and planting, and tending and harvesting produce.

The NYU Urban Farm Lab's genesis required navigating city and university bureaucracy in an era of skepticism over growing food in city spaces. In the mid-2000s, when graduate student Daniel Bowman Simon approached us about using a grassy space adjacent to NYU faculty housing for an urban garden, the food studies faculty was enthused and, having discussed such an idea for years, regarded his initiative as a welcome catalyst. University administration, however, was not sure it wanted to take on the project. Pessimistic though logical questions ensued. Them: *What about rats?* Us: *There will always be rats.* Them: *Won't the grounds look ugly in the winter?* Us: *A dormant garden in winter might look "ugly" to those used to a manicured lawn aesthetic, but it is part of understanding sustainable and healthy food systems.* Them: *Isn't the soil contaminated?* Us: *No, we had it checked multiple times.* Them: *Who is going to fund it?* Us: *Mmm, we'll figure that out* (we did). Them: *Will anyone be interested?* Us: *We have overwhelming support from NYU faculty, students, and staff and the broader community. We'll create a hands-on class that will be a hit with students* (it is).

The idea of an on-campus garden had long been a goal, as at the time, urban gardens were an important emerging presence all over the United States (and globally) in urban metropolises and on college campuses as part of sustainability initiatives. One of us (Jennifer) had already been sponsoring small student garden plots. Building on that experience, we, with assistance from Marion Nestle, applied for and received an NYU sustainability grant. Before any planting could begin, however, there were months of negotiation and eventual approval from the Greenwich Village Community Board and the NYC Landmarks Commission (the plot of land fell within the landmarked Silver Towers complex between Bleecker and Houston Streets). In time, NYU realized the importance (in material and also public relations terms) of participating in the endeavor and soon proved a supportive partner, providing material assistance with the landscaping and soil requirements and helping shepherd the plans through bureaucratic challenges. The benefit of green spaces in urban areas is well documented, as is the health benefit of participating in growing and cooking food. In addition, the Urban Farm Lab fosters a camaraderie that creates and strengthens community. There are many more benefits.

Along with our Kitchen Food Lab (another important experiential learning space), the Urban Farm Lab serves as an event space, auxiliary classroom, research site, and community hub. Reinforcing theoretical discussions on organic farming, sustainable practices, Indigenous techniques, global and heirloom crops, and mitigating food waste, the Urban Farm Lab allows us to get our hands dirty (literally and figuratively) while we align theory and practice. Our urban agriculture courses are remarkably popular and open to all NYU students, across NYU divisions and schools, majors and academic levels. Graduate food studies students pose research projects, including investigating the economic viability of ancient grains, comparative composting strategies, water restriction and catchment, companion crop paring, and trellis design. Most recently, we added a mushroom cultivation project and mycology research, as well as a seed-saving library. Student groups such as the Food and Racial Equity Collective and the Food Policy Alliance tend their own plots and hold public talks and events on site. Our robust study abroad program discussed above has plots for each course, allowing students to explore specific seeds native to the regions they traveled. The Urban Farm Lab works in concert with our teaching Kitchen Lab, growing specific crops needed for the food production courses, while organic kitchen scraps return to the Urban Farm Lab for composting. We work with neighboring food outreach organizations by donating all excess harvested produce. Finally, during the COVID-19 pandemic, the Urban Farm Lab served as an important outdoor oasis (while adhering to social distancing and masking requirements).

Public Programming and Collaborative Knowledge Creation
Amy Bentley

In addition to my more conventionally scholarly research, I have become increasingly involved in projects and platforms that encourage engagement with the general public. In addition to providing an educational space, the projects invite and are dependent on others' ideas and materials, which results in the co-creation of knowledge. The two ventures discussed here are the Experimental Cuisine Collective (2007–16) and the Food and COVID-19 NYC Digital Archive and Collection.

The Experimental Cuisine Collective (ECC) began as an idea hatched by NYU chemistry professor Kent Kirshenbaum, NYC modernist cuisine chef Will Goldfarb, and me. We sought to create a public-facing group that could explore the intersection of food and science in a way that differed from traditional food science. After enlisting NYU food studies doctoral student Anne McBride (now vice president of programs at the James Beard Foundation), we fostered a diverse group of scholars, scientists, chefs, writers, journalists, performance artists, teachers, and food enthusiasts for monthly meetings on diverse topics. Our overall aim was to develop a broad-based and rigorous academic approach that employed techniques and approaches from the humanities, arts, and sciences to examine the properties, boundaries, and conventions of food, explored food and science vis-à-vis aesthetics, historical, and cultural notions, and that above all celebrated taste and deliciousness.

Topics included a study of the chemical properties of seaweed, the science of chocolate chip cookies, experiments with sous vide, among many others. We envisioned the ECC, which received recognition in *Time Magazine* for its innovative approach to food education, as filling a gap in the current landscape of food-focused organizations and public discourse on food. While there were many organizations that emphasized organics, local food, or culinary tourism, none explored the intersection of food and science in a way that was different from traditional food science programs and industries. We wanted to highlight and elevate science as applied to craft and creative (non-industry) enterprise. There was an emerging science-averse approach to food, and we wanted to show how science was a profound part of all types of interactions and manipulations of food. Other meeting topics included the science of umami, Japanese pickling traditions, cheese and microbial communities, and food, soil, and sustainable urban design. The popular monthly meetings ran for a decade until we needed to turn our attention to other projects. Happily, by that time (2016), there were other organizations that had emerged in this space, which made the decision easier.

However, in 2024 we launched a new iteration of ECC programming in close collaboration with the James Beard Foundation.

In contrast to the ECC's public forums and workshops, the Food and COVID-19 NYC Digital Archive and Collection lives entirely online and sprang from a graduate seminar forced to make a dramatic pandemic pivot. By early March 2020, it became clear that my Food History graduate seminar would undergo some drastic changes, including by becoming entirely remote. It soon felt inappropriate to continue with the class as if nothing extraordinary, and extraordinarily scary, was happening. Because COVID was unavoidable, and in part because it felt false not to somehow grapple with it in our class, I gave students the option to use class assignments to write and think about the pandemic academically. Eventually, I came to understand these food and COVID assignments—which were not only written essays but also photo essays and blog posts—as capturing in real time this momentous era. I began to frame and discuss these assignments as data: historical evidence to serve as artifacts for a future public that wanted to know about New Yorkers' experiences, such as what they thought about and what they ate, during this global pandemic when their city was in lockdown (Bentley and Borkowsky, 2020).

These assignments became the base of the Food and COVID-19 NYC Digital Archive and Collection. With the assistance of graduate student Stephanie Borkowsky, we collected any and all related materials: photos, personal narratives, menus, media articles, and more. We invited the general public to upload their materials as well. What began in the spring of 2020 as a NYU food studies graduate seminar class project had evolved into a space capturing the food experiences of New Yorkers as they navigated the traumas of the COVID-19 pandemic through 2020 and into the spring of 2021. While the ongoing pandemic will affect NYC food for years, this archive documents a full year, from March 2020 through March 2021. Following the ebbs and flows of the pandemic's intensity, the site captures the landscape of food topically (food insecurity, restaurants, shopping, and at home) as well as chronologically. The project is contextualized with introductory and framing essays, timelines, links to other similar collections, related newsletters and blogs. Thus, the space functions as much as a clearinghouse of information and interpretive virtual museum site as it is an archive for raw data. While we have stopped actively collecting documents, anyone can upload materials, and it is a space for researchers now and into the future.

REFERENCES

Allison, Noah, Krishnendu Ray, and Jaclyn Rohel. 2021. "Mobilizing the Streets: The Role of Food Vendors in Urban Life." *Food, Culture, and Society* 24 (1): 2–14. https://doi.org/10.1080/15528014.2020.1860454.

Bachórz, Agata, and Fabio Parasecoli. 2020. "Why Should We Care? Two Experiences in the Politics of Food and Food Research." *Ethnologia Polona* 41:13–31. doi:10.23858/ethp.2020.41.2301.

Banaji, Jairus. 2020. *A Brief History of Commercial Capitalism*. Chicago: Haymarket.

Bentley, Amy, and Stephanie Borkowsky. 2020. "The Food and COVID-19 NYC Archive: Mapping the Pandemic's Effect on Food in Real Time." *Gastronomica* 20, no. 4 (December): 8–11. https://doi.org/10.1525/gfc.2020.20.4.8.

Chaudhuri, Supriya. 2020. "View: The Working Person's Right to Life." *Economic Times*, May 12. https://m.economictimes.com.

Chevalier, Jacques M., and Daniel J. Buckles. 2019. *Participatory Action Research: Theory and Methods for Engaged Inquiry*. New York: Routledge.

Datta, Dilip. "Women at Work." 2020. *Statesman News Service*, December 8. https://www.thestatesman.com.

De Certeau, Michel. 1984. *The Practice of Everyday Life*. Translated by Steven Rendall. Berkeley: University of California Press.

Economic Times. 2020, April 23. "Lockdown in India Has Impacted 40 Million Internal Migrants: World Bank." https://economictimes.indiatimes.com.

Experimental Cuisine Collective. 2007–16. https://experimentalcuisine.com/.

Gordon Da Cruz, Cynthia. 2018. "Community-Engaged Scholarship: Toward a Shared Understanding of Practice." *The Review of Higher Education* 41 (2): 147–67.

International Labour Organization. 2017. "Persisting Servitude and Gradual Shifts Towards Recognition and Dignity of Labour. A Study of Employers of Domestic Workers in Delhi and Mumbai." https://www.ilo.org.

———. 2022. "About Domestic Work." https://www.ilo.org.

Kumar, Arun. 2020. "How the Lack of Reliable Data Hurts the Most Vulnerable Indians." *Scroll.in*, September 16. https://scroll.in.

Manzini, Enzo. 2015. *Design, When Everybody Designs. An Introduction to Design for Social Innovation*. Cambridge, MA: MIT Press.

Nath, Damini. 2020. "Govt. Has No Data of Migrant Workers' Death, Loss of Job." *Hindu.com*, September 14. https://www.thehindu.com.

New York University. (2020). Food and COVID-19 NYC Digital Archive and Collection. https://wp.nyu.edu/foodandcovid19/.

RoyChowdhury, Supriya. *City of Shadows. Slums and Informal Work in Bangalore*. Cambridge, UK: Cambridge University Press.

Sanyal, Kalyan. 2014. *Rethinking Capitalist Development*. New Delhi: Routledge.

Street Vendor Project. n.d. Advisory Board. Accessed January 20, 2022. http://street-vendor.org/about-us-2/advisory-board/.

Warde, Alan. 2014. "After Taste: Culture, Consumption and Theories of Practice." *Journal of Consumer Culture* 14 (3): 279–303. https://doi.org/10.1177/146954051454782.

———. 2016. *The Practice of Eating*. Cambridge, UK: Polity.

Yamunan, Sruthisagar. 2020. "As Supreme Court Fails to Protect Migrant Workers' Rights, High Courts Show the Way." *Scroll.in*, May 18. https://scroll.in/.

14

In Closing

Knowledge-Production in Institutional Context

KRISHNENDU RAY

In the introductory chapter, Fabio Parasecoli and Amy Bentley opened with a question: What is food studies at NYU? They went on to illustrate divergent attitudes of faculty and students to discipline and method. In the process, they underlined that what we call food studies is built in close proximity to the social sciences, such as economics, and the health sciences, such as nutrition, dietetics, and public health. That proximity makes us different from a purely humanities discipline attuned to critique as theoretical knowledge. We are as oriented to pragmatics—what levers to pull to make it a more just world—as to positive knowledge, which is shaped by actionable, albeit contingent, information and concepts compared to pure critique. If we were in a wholly humanities or a social science department, we would have been different from our current public humanities and public social science positioning. That is probably the most important insight of this book: our topics, perspective, methods, and episteme, as a whole, are decisively shaped by our institutional location and posture toward modes of knowledge-production and dissemination. Although that is true of all programs, the fact that we have to communicate and make collective decisions with our colleagues in the hard social sciences and the biological sciences, rare for a typical humanities program, makes us more self-conscious of it. Location matters to knowledge production, and we have been elbowed by and have elbowed our way into our current location (Abbott 2001, 1999).

A Genesis: People, Place, Affiliations

Marion Nestle founded NYU food studies between 1988 and 2003 by trading the hospitality program with another school (NYU is a network of about a dozen quasi-autonomous institutions called schools). She moved decisively away from home economics, entangling herself with restaurant consultants and colleagues in organizations such as the Old-ways Preservation and Exchange Trust, a gathering of chefs, food writers, and health and environmental scholars. She belongs to a constellation of outsiders who became public intellectuals because of the academy's weakness at producing actionable critique in accessible language; we see that as an important task in producing knowledge for strengthening democracies. I see Nestle in the tradition of Rachel Carson, Vandana Shiva, Alice Waters, Joan Dye Gussow, and Janet Poppendieck. The NYU food studies program still exhibits that kind of attention to the public. Nestle sought to mimic Boston University's gastronomy program but withstood the criticism from Alice Waters about avoiding farmers and agriculturalists, only by conceding to her critique in the long run. Soon after NYU food studies obtained state approval, Marian Burros, a *New York Times* food writer, provided the first blast of publicity, which we have always been privileged to get due to our location in this mon-strously churning media market called New York City. Nestle says that *New York Times* coverage filled the classroom when the doors opened in 1996, and the rest is history.

This is of course a recent history written by the winners. There were those who opposed and disagreed with that move. Some of them be-came chairs after Marion Nestle stepped down and shaped the program in other ways. There were those who never got over the removal of the hospitality program, as you have seen in Jon Deutsch's essay. Food stud-ies was the product of a particular persona in interaction with the local environment, at a particular historical moment, grabbing what she could to build what she could, according to her current conception and network. If all this had happened at the end of the previous century, we would have been a home economics department, which the department was through most of the twentieth century. There are still subterranean traces of that prehistory in the building, with the old-style "home ec" kitchens and sewing machines stacked away that Nestle speaks of in her essay, most prominently the significance of a cohort of white women, in spite of the slowly changing demographics. Our naming of the Food Lab and Urban Farm Lab are not that far from the anxieties of home economics. Sometime in the future, after we are all dead, someone will write the real history of the program. For now, we will have to do with this first draft.

People on the ground with particular training and perspective help shape an institution's personality and positioning. Two people were decisive in turning Nestle's grand vision into a working model: Amy Bentley, the historian and American studies scholar, and Jennifer Berg, a product of the hotel school at Cornell University. Someone had to implement, correct, and nudge Nestle's grand but thinly populated vision, and it was this dynamic duo who decisively shaped the content and the character of the program. Bentley did that with her historical training, which helped facilitate a humanities orientation rather than a hospitality or an agriculture program. If that first hire had been an agricultural economist, as we hired much later, the program would have looked more like the Cornell nutrition program or the University of Vermont Department of Nutrition and Food Science, with its food systems program, than what it looks like today. In fact, that hire bifurcated the program into a nutrition program and a food studies program. History was embedded into the DNA of the department. Gender got written into the content and style of doing food studies. Bentley's work on World War II food rationing and victory gardens, baby food, and women's work strengthened what was the nutrition department's "female centered aura and culture." It also decisively linked us to the pragmatics of raising children, supporting partners, and taking care of other lives, which someone like me benefitted from immensely when I was left to raise a child on my own.

Berg, on the other hand, ran everything. She still does. By the time this book goes to press, she will be the chair of the department, formally leading what she has built at least by half. Berg brought attention to the food business and entrepreneurship side, in spite of abandoning the name hospitality, perhaps related to her own prehistory where the Cornell hospitality program was disdained by the Cornell hotel school. We all have our rotten histories to deal with. She ran everything and brought breathless energy in some directions and finesse in others. She was overworked and kept an unrelenting pace. It is because of her that the NYU food studies program has survived over the last three decades, and she did it while pursuing her own doctorate in the program, graduating as one of the earliest food studies PhDs. She brought style to a bumbling group of academics who could not distinguish grape variety or cheese type to save their lives. There is still the Berg law of never serving cubed cheeses at departmental functions. Caterers have lost jobs over that rule. She taught us how to be classy by acquiring the cultural capital we never had but needed to survive in the big city. We would have been eaten alive without her. She worked, and she worked, and she worked, with an ambitious leader and not very practical colleagues.

Bentley and Berg tied the early growth of the program to the trajectory of the Association for the Study of Food and Society (ASFS), a group that attracted scholars primarily working on food consumption from around the United States and Canada, mostly from the humanities and the soft social sciences, and the Agriculture, Food and Human Values Society, which attracted scholars working on agricultural production and distribution. This connected the food studies program, otherwise isolated, to larger, productive networks of scholars, editors, and teachers. Many of us involved ourselves in this organization chaperoning it for decades, serving as president, vice president, editing the journal *Food, Culture & Society* and running its treasury. ASFS gave intellectual and organizational heft to a puny sapling planted in the dog-eat-dog world of American academia, with a superstar chair and meager resources. It is still a small program of five to six full time faculty.

Quantitative and Qualitative Research

Most scholars know what quantitative research is. It is often conducted with large datasets—as Juan Herrera shows with 5,981 recipes with 557 unique ingredients and James Malin demonstrates with 5,666 articles and 11,678 keywords—using mathematical tools, to make generalizable arguments, here about the sources of taste and modes of analysis and more usually about the nature and cause of illness, wellness, and inequalities. It is mostly quantitative scholars who think of ethnographic, small-n survey, archival and design work as qualitative research. For our quantitative and objectivist colleagues, we are at best doing a science of subjectivity and intersubjectivity. Sometimes, the mutual characterization tends toward incompatibility. In other institutional locations, we may not have to characterize ourselves as qualitative researchers, but in our department, we do, although some of us—Carolyn Dimitri, Beth Weitzman, and Juan C. S. Herrera—use quantitative methods as well. In that sense, NYU food studies is closer to cultural sociology, which finds both quantitative and qualitative work acceptable, rather than cultural anthropology, where ethnographic methods are de rigueur. We work with aptitude, affinity, and skill for one or the other kind of symbolic work—with words or numbers—but it is possible to do a PhD in our department using either of those tools. In the case of Herrera, we had to draw in a physicist from the engineering school to help him construct his network science tools, which even our in-house quantitative economist was unwilling to embark on. We wrestled over whether the project was more amenable to a stringent quantitative or qualitative analysis, and he had both skills (partly because of his training as an economist in Colombia). On the other hand, Grace Choi and Fabio Parasecoli approach recipes using ethnographic methods and design thinking. Working with a handful of dishes, Choi seeks to deliver the affective and sensory investment of the video game in designing a recipe, showing how recipes serve denotative purpose and connotative function, where much has to be left unsaid. She underlines the challenge of converting actions to words and back to action again. What is gained and what is lost in those transformations? Analogously, Parasecoli asks, How can the space between the hand and the head be turned into an opportunity to build toward a possible future? That is probably the most enduring question shaping our program. Eric Himmelfarb extends that challenge to the relationship between the aesthetic, the ethical, and the pedagogical. His teaching represents the process by which "the ordinary juice of prose" is turned into "the strong wine of poetry" through the intermediation of activism. As you can see from the topics, we are quite ecumenical about our subject and our methods.

We accept PhD students with a wider array of methodological skills than most of us experienced in our own doctoral trajectories. But like all good things, there is a limit. At what point does doing too many things lead to doing many things poorly, where depth is sacrificed for breadth? We have to figure that out. We are protected now by the fact that we are a miniscule PhD program admitting one funded student a year and graduating one every few years. We like it to be small so that we do not offload too many graduates into the marketplace.

Public Audiences and Private Protections

We think of the public in two forms: policy-making/policy-changing and as the locus of popular culture. Nestle, Dimitri, and Weitzman deal more directly with advising public institutions in formulating policies or NGOs in changing laws. Most of the work, for the rest of us, is a mix of interventions in policy making, advocacy, and popular culture. From Marion Nestle down, our public policy posture makes us critical of the profit motive, especially monopoly profits and market-distorting accumulation, but we are not anti-private property or anti-market per se, which we think are important resources counterbalancing the weight of the state and monopoly capital. Markets predate capitalism, and most markets are out of its reach. In that sense, our understanding of historical capitalism is Braudelian, as a particularly modern relationship between large capital, finance, and the state (Braudel 1992). In her short piece toward the end of the book, Carolyn Dimitri shows us how to work with market regulations and socially useful standards like the National Organic Standards Board to shift resources toward conservation and sustainability in the Farm Bill, triangulating producer, consumer, and public interests while keeping the environment in view. In that sense, we are closer to the perspectives of Thomas Piketty, Kate Raworth, and Amartya Sen than with wholesale anti-market critics. We are critical of neoliberal capitalism, but we have also learned the big lesson of the twentieth century, which is that the destruction of markets and small properties—as happened in the state-oriented collectivization drives in the Soviet Union and in China—are catastrophic not only to agrarian production and consumption but to democratic institutions. They have also led to the biggest famines of the twentieth century (just as liberal colonialism led to the biggest famines of the nineteenth century; see Davis 2017; Sen 2001). Dimitri puts it most clearly when she writes, "I am an applied economist and have a strong belief in markets." What Dimitri states clearly, many of us follow in practice (although not uniformly). Importantly, we, unlike neoliberals, do not consider markets and property to be sacred. We approach such things as potentially better managed for social purposes. As Piketty (2020) argues, proprietary ideologies have an emancipatory dimension if we do not go to excesses of sacralizing them. Partly because there are few alternatives to markets in processing information about supply and demand and diluting the totalitarian power of the state (as the twentieth century showed; see Sen 2001). We have over time developed an appreciation of the necessary balance among the weight of the state, the market, and civic organizations, along with the necessity of privacy for individuals, households, and voluntary associations (a privacy that has historically protected the lives and bodies of women and gender fluid persons). As a result, most of us find ourselves on the liberal end of the social democratic spectrum in our conception and work, shaped by the history of Marxism and poststructuralism but neither Marxists nor poststructuralists. That is a different trajectory from radical relativists.

From Poetry to Policy

In spite of the occasional reference to the magically productive conceptualization of epistemic relativists such as Bruno Latour (2004), who has done wonders for science and technology studies, we occupy a different part of the current knowledge production universe. Doing science, we think, is a different project from doing science studies. Science studies is a monologue against the emic triumphalism of modern science. Epistemic relativism holds that all methods that produce facts, concepts, and evidence are equally legitimate in their historical and social contexts and that there are no ways to distinguish the efficacy of one over the other in particular socio-temporal moments. Their exemplary technique is the use of the ethnographic present tense. Rare exceptions in our department are hard epistemic relativists; most appear to believe that some modes of constructing facts and deploying evidence for arguments prove to be superior over time; the analogous technique here is historicism (after Bourdieu 2004; Oreskes 2019; Piketty 2022). That most of us are progressives is not because we are better social scientists but because we come later in history and hence have the privilege of hindsight. Our attitude toward science is closer in spirit to the closing lines of Rachel Carson's *Silent Spring*: "It is our alarming misfortune that so primitive a science has armed itself with the most modern and terrible weapons, and that in turning them against the insects it has also turned them against the earth" (1962, 297). Our epistemic orientation is post-Latourian (having learned much from him, such as his critique of critique, the uncertainty, and the ratio of pragmatics and power at the heart of the scientific enterprise), working toward a better science and a limited one (see Oreskes 2019), all of it socially constructed, but with different efficacy, judged in hindsight, rather than cultivating equal doubt about all forms of knowledge at the moment of their construction.

Let me illustrate our positioning with an example borrowed from Tom Scott-Smith's recent book *On an Empty Stomach* (2020, 106–20). On the way to the doctor's office, a patient feels weak and bloated, with edema, swollen stomach, thickened skin, hair with reddish tinge. He can barely keep up with his mother. The doctor examines him. Runs a few simple tests, including a middle under arm circumference with a special tape measure, and diagnoses him with kwashiorker, first named in 1933 on the Gold Coast of Africa. In a sense, on the way to the doctor's office, the patient feels ill; on the way back, he gets a disease, specifically a disease of protein deficiency. In the pursuit of protein, you can also witness the emergence of "nutritionism," where hunger is turned into the need for protein (Scrinis 2013). Hunger, in this case, is medicalized, as Foucault would have put it in *The Birth of a Clinic* (1976), turned into the need for a specific nutrient rather than for food in general, which turns out to be a disease of poverty. Furthermore, it turns out that this long persistent but newly "discovered" disease by Westerners drives the search for the delivery of various manufactured, for-profit nutrients—dehydrated liver, desiccated gut, Marmite, cod liver oil, and so on—on the back of colonial power. Here knowledge is linked to colonialism. A social problem of inequality is turned into a logistical problem of supplying the right nutrient to the right person in the colony with the help of colonialism, by people who claim to know better. That could be a Foucauldian analysis par excellence.

A dietitian or an intervention nutritionist would need to do something for the hungry patient in front of her. The patient needs to be fed—not too much and not too suddenly, and if possible, he needs to be temporarily removed from the chronic condition of poverty. Rarely would the dietitian know how to challenge the unequal economic structures that keep people poor on the Gold Coast. It is an altogether different order of problem from critically analyzing hunger. Marion Nestle's attempt, among others, has been to move dietitians to see the larger context without changing their profession. In that sense, she is closer to food studies than to dietetics, which, like a physician, focuses primarily on singular patients. The relationship of the dietitian and the patient is one of providing succor and aid in healing, not to provide a critical analysis of inequality. For the patient, a consultation with a sociologist would be the wrong prescription at this point. That is the source of perpetual tension and mutual incomprehension between the two programs in our department. Some of it is productive, some obstructive. Our undergraduate curriculum wrestles most directly with this tension. Stephanie Rogus's chapter shows the attempt to develop a civic dietetics within the profession, especially after 1997, that is culturally attuned and attentive to questions of sustainability. She represents the capacity to acquire qualitative depth while not abandoning quantitative generalizability. She also shows the uses of reduction without being reductionist, which is an important lesson to humanists who tend to panic when confronted with the necessity of reduction, which is essential if we are to speak, write, teach, or intervene in the world. Most importantly, she highlights professional developments in putting the patient in context while providing succor and aid in healing, by way of one-on-one interventions. We can willingly switch from critical to pragmatic tasks in our academic work, as we do in other aspects of our life.

More broadly, in our estimation, there are numerous ways to deal with the problem of hunger. Medicalization of chronic scarcity can help in healing and should be considered a legitimate way to intervene in the world, at least as legitimate as providing a critical theoretical intervention. That becomes clearer in the case of leprosy, which has some of the highest incidence rates in India, Brazil, and Indonesia. According to modern biomedicine, it is a disease caused by a bacterial infection and not a curse or the result of moral deviation (according to numerous vernacular understandings of disease and disability). It is often associated with poverty, malnutrition, and overcrowding, resulting in an opportunistic infection. But it can be treated, quite easily, in fact, with antibiotics over a three month period and cured, saving the patient from the deformity, pain and social ostracization that goes with leaving leprosy untreated. It is better if the problem is medicalized rather than socialized (which it has been through much of its history), with all its long durable prejudices, isolation, and painful, debilitating death. We know from modern biomedicine and statistical analysis that 95 percent of people have natural immunity to the bacillus (CDC 2022). Those two facts are used by the WHO, after renaming it as Hansen's disease, to make a dent in widespread social prejudice against the patients so that the disease itself can be diagnosed, treated, and eradicated. This kind of open-mindedness about the nature of knowledge and intervention is not only realistic and helpful but also generates humility about instituted ways of knowing and doing in our world, some of which may not be our ways of doing things. Clinical interventions are at least as important as refinement of theories about science and society. And specialists matter. Furthermore, not all methods and argumentation and rules of evidence are equally salient or suspect. Those kinds of judgments need specification in each case. These examples—Kwashiorker and Hansen's—also point to the slow transition in food studies away from its unbearably quaint Euro-Americanisms that have shaped its birth in rich, consumer societies.

Our perspective of taking specialists seriously, in medicine to history writing, in spite of legitimate critiques of science and expert knowledge, has been shaped by the hijacking of skepticism by right-wing nationalists in a wide range of places such as India, Brazil, and the United States of America. That has had a deleterious impact on the profession of history writing, too. For instance, nativists and untrained Hindu nationalists are rewriting India's history to erase the contribution of Muslims and other minorities. So, our epistemic politics is strategic and contextual, alive to the contemporary challenges of revanchist nationalisms.

As a result, we are equally likely to ask the questions that Beth Weitzman does: "How can public policies be used to improve the health and well-being of . . . people, especially for those communities with greatest needs?," as we would pose queries by scholars in the humanities: "What is scientific knowledge and how has it been historically constituted?" Our work resides mostly at midlevel conception and execution in the social sciences and the humanities, rather than meta-level ontological and epistemic queries. Our location forces us to act in spite of our doubts. For instance, we are quite sure that smoking is deleterious to health, notwithstanding all the epistemic uncertainty about causation that surrounded it and was spread by cigarette companies, which is another example used in this book. There is also enough evidence that drinking too much soda undermines wellness, notwithstanding other issues of the autonomy of poor people (as with cigarettes) in regulating soda consumption. In contrast, there is very good evidence to show that a robust infrastructure of clean, piped water and separate waste disposal is probably the most important positive interventions in the lives of poor people globally, in spite of its dangers of governmentality (Banerjee and Duflo 2011, 68). That is a function of the modern centralized state and can be attributed to thinking like one. Nevertheless it is a good thing to recommend, given what we know today. We try not to wrestle with excessive doubt or considerations of complexity in that case. Of course, like Latour, we are sure that nothing can be said with certainty until after the fact, but an immediate and pragmatic perspective does not allow us the theoretical leisure of total doubt at a particular moment. What we believe to be true and egalitarian might in the long-run turn out to be inadequately so, but we are willing to take that risk to act in the world today. We might have to change our mind, once more evidence comes in. Our difference with radical epistemic relativists is twofold: the temporal horizon and task orientation. The temporality of epistemic relativists is the historical present. At a particular moment, all there is to scientific query is doubt and various socially constituted strategies to break through them. Our temporal horizon, in the department, is like social scientists, over the medium-run and across historical periods, where there can be greater certainty. Secondly, our task is often positive, in contrast to critique. We seek to make something, to build something materially, or symbolically, with words, numbers. and actions. The task of pure critique might be the pleasure of intellection, the delight of distanced cognition, which is precisely what drives Jon Duetsch to distraction as you have seen earlier and as I will address below.

The logic of acting now is pushed by our colleagues in nutrition and public health. That is the reason we embraced and encouraged others, for instance, during the COVID-19 pandemic, to take the available vaccines, not because we were certain of their consequences in the long run but because we were convinced of their current efficacy, given expert knowledge based on double-blind, quantitative, and generalizable studies, at that moment of decision-making. That impulse can be extended to supporting public health initiatives, providing nutrition advice in spite of a million uncertainties and complexities, or mounting an exhibition on food in the city. That is also the reason we are much more open to the uses of expert knowledge than those more strongly motivated by radical epistemic doubt. Power is entangled with knowledge, as Michel Foucault demonstrated, both in the restrictive sense and in its productive elaboration of subjectivities, but for us, domination may not be fatally intertwined with each and every form of knowing and acting in the world. Here we are closer to Pierre Bourdieu's techniques of epistemic reflexivity in separating the object of analysis from spontaneous prenotions (see Bourdieu 2004; Steinmetz 2022). That is how we avoid the paralysis of pure critique and are willing to risk intervening in the world today. Others in more humanities-oriented departments could be elaborating on much deeper epistemic doubt, but that is not the nature of the game specific to our location.

Jon Deutsch, both a product and a critic of the NYU food studies program, poses the question sharply from the other direction: Should we be making a better banana ice cream (to take his example)? How far can we go in the direction of doing and attending to immediacy without becoming unrecognizable as a program in the social sciences and the humanities? In fact, in food studies, we are better suited to serve James Malin's hunger for the opposite, his quest to learn *"about* food, *about* cooking, or *about* restaurants" rather than the actual execution of a dish. There are lots of terrific hospitality and food science programs in the United States, and as Marion Nestle notes in her chapter, she exchanged that kind of program for food studies. Nevertheless, we are still trying to find that sweet spot between systematic critical analysis and intervention, without becoming a program for product development. It is unlikely that NYU food studies will become an alternative food lab comparable to the Drexel enterprise. We see ourselves in a different corner within the ecology of specialized institutions, such as at Syracuse University (with greater attention to system) or the University of Toronto's program (with its strength in history), but one without an extensive food science curriculum (beyond the undergraduate level).

It is worth underlining here that although we work adjacent to nutritionists, the food studies degree is not a degree in nutrition. Lisa Sasson's work with dysphagia patients and students is shaped by her biography and proximity to food studies, but her specialization in dietetics is separate and different from the scope and nature of research in food studies. We contain ourselves to the subject matter and methods of the social sciences and the humanities, not the sciences such as nutrition and dietetics. Those are different degrees housed in the same department. That is why we think recognition of specialization is important and that different departments working with food within differing institutional ecologies should do different things. The University of Vermont program, for instance, is closer to food science than ours. These differences between programs is one reason among many that food studies is unlikely to become a discipline any time soon. We do not bring the degree of cohesion and abstraction to the project of studying food in the social world, and others such as cultural anthropology and sociology are already engaged in that task. We learn from them, we work with them, and sometimes we contest them from our location, but we have no ambition or wish or capacity to replace them. We do not think we need another discipline. And sometimes it is good to develop a view from outside disciplines to grasp their limits better. It spares us the defensive and wasteful boundary drawing that is central to every discipline making.

Eating, the anthropologist Annamarie Mol (2021, 100) shows, escapes the clear bifurcation between willful choices and natural processes. As a result, she celebrates doing as tinkering, making do—like Luce Giard (1998) taught us long ago—trying again and again and again to do a little better, exemplified by everyday cooking. Eating, on which survival depends, is an act of cultivation, both in the agricultural sense and the consuming sense, of trying, facing defeat and trying again. That is our approach in building a food studies program, curriculum, and training for our students, in collaboration with others in other disciplines and locations, in our university, and in other universities elsewhere in the world.

Cooking Slowly, Blooming Late: Public Scholarship and Pedagogy Driven Approach

In Marion Nestle's recent autobiography, *Slow Cooked* (2022), she tells a version of our program's founding. She shows us how and why she came to her career late. That temporal slowness can also be attributed to the program she institutionalized. Despite the youthfulness of a number of contributors in this collection, the nature of the multidisciplinary work entails a longer takeoff because it demands mastery of many fields. From Marion Nestle onward—all the professors in our program are close to their sixties—you will find us cooking slowly and blooming late. Part of this is a function of our inexact fit with the disciplines we were trained in. Part of it is linked to the institutional wandering we did in our lives. Part of it was the burden of caregiving that often took decades of our lives to get on track before we could concentrate on the profession. Almost all of us like to cook and do cook regularly with degrees of obligation and pleasure. That takes time and commitment. When I first came to the department, that was one of its most inviting aspects. We were encouraged to bring our children, pets, and partners to work. We often ate together at work. You can get a feel for that kind of inter-twining of career and care-work in Grace Choi's writing about cradling her daughter's bottom in one hand while reaching for the principle of voice-narrated, hands-free recipes. As James Malin notes astutely, there is much in common between research and cooking: techniques take time and discipline, traditions dominate, "It is never over, never perfect, and never complete." As we grew bigger and became more professional, some of those practices fell by the wayside, but we avoided mercenary competition and petty jealousies that are the bane of so many good departments. That takes a certain kind of mindset and a certain horizon of possibility, where academic work is one of the dimensions of our social assessment of each other. Careers are important, so are children, partners, parents, pets, along with social advocacy and activism. As we lay down some lines of inquiry and tracks of investigation and intervention, we are hoping to reduce the age of academic performance in this corner of a multidisciplinary field.

Compared to the departments many of us have graduated from, at NYU food studies, teaching often drives a substantial part of the research and publication. Recall the student who encouraged Beth Weitzman to engage with the semiotics of calorie labeling, or Lisa Sasson's students reflecting on their body image; the NYU Urban Farm Lab instigated by Daniel Bowman Simon and cultivated by the Food and Racial Equity Collective; the Experimental Cuisine Collective nurtured by Anne Mc-Bride; and the Food and COVID-19 Digital Archive nursed by Stephanie Borkowsky, as shown by Amy Bentley. Analogously, Alex Jimerson, a Hodinöšönih student of ours, belonging to the Wolf Clan of the Seneca

Nation, had noted to me long before I had read theories of interspecies entanglement, "My garden is coming along nicely except I ran into some problems with the Squash Vine Borer which took out a couple of my plants. It always hurts when you lose a plant but just have to remember it's a learning process and we've got to share what we grow even if it's not with our human relatives." That transformed my thinking long before I read Annemarie Mol's *Eating in Theory* (2021) or Merlin Sheldrake's *Entangled Life* (2020). Our students' ways of studying, understanding, and at times intervening in the world forces us to reconsider our own goals as teachers and researchers. Most importantly, each new recruit—faculty and student—has to be retrained to circumvent the mutual epistemic disdain between the sciences, social sciences, and the humanities, which is second nature in most disciplines, and they have to learn to be more ecumenical, less proselytizing, as they grapple with the tools, substance, and arguments for food studies.

REFERENCES

Abbott, Andrew. 1999. *Department and Discipline*. Chicago: University of Chicago Press.
———. 2001. *Chaos of Disciplines*. Chicago: University of Chicago Press.
Banerjee, Abhijit V., and Esther Duflo. 2011. *Poor Economics. A Radical Rethinking of the Way to Fight Global Poverty*. New York: Public Affairs.
Bourdieu, Pierre. 2004. *Science of Science and Reflexivity*. Chicago: University of Chicago Press.
Braudel, Fernand. 1992. *Civilization and Capitalism, 15th-18th Century*. 3 vols. Berkeley: University of California Press.
Bridle, James. 2022. *Ways of Being. Animals, Plants, Machines: Planetary Intelligence*. New York: Farrer, Strauss & Giroux.
Carson, Rachel. 1962. *Silent Spring*. Boston: Mariner Books.
Center for Disease Control (CDC). 2021. *World Leprosy Day: Bust the Myths, Learn the Facts*. https://www.cdc.gov.
Davis, Mike. 2017. *Late Victorian Holocausts. El Niño Famines and the Making of the Third World*. London: Verso.
Giard, Luce, ed., with Michel de Certeau and Pierre Mayol. 1998. *Practice of Everyday Life*. Vol. 2, *Living and Cooking*. Minneapolis: University of Minnesota Press.
Foucault, Michel. 1976. *The Birth of a Clinic: An Archaeology of Medical Perception*. London: Tavistock.
Fukuyama, Francis. 2022. *Liberalism and its Discontents*. New York: Farrar, Straus and Giroux.
Graeber, David, and David Wengrow. 2021. *The Dawn of Everything*. New York: Farrar, Straus and Giroux.

Latour, Bruno. 2004. "Why Has Critique Run Out of Steam? From Matters of Fact to Matters of Concern." *Critical Inquiry* 30, no. 2 (Winter): 225–48.

Mol, Annemarie. 2021. *Eating in Theory*. Durham, NC: Duke University Press.

Nestle, Marion. 2022. *Slow Cooked*. Berkeley: University of California Press.

Oreskes, Naomi. 2019. *Why Trust Science?* Princeton, NJ: Princeton University Press.

Piketty, Thomas. 2020. *Capital and Ideology*. Cambridge, MA: Belknap, Harvard University Press.

———. 2022. *A Brief History of Equality*. Cambridge, MA: Harvard University Press.

Rowat, Kate. 2017. *Doughnut Economics: Seven Ways to Think like a 21st-Century Economist*. New York: Chelsea Green.

Scrinis, Gyorgy. 2013. *Nutritionism: The Science and Politics of Dietary Advice*. New York: Columbia University Press

Sen, Amartya. 2000. *Development as Freedom*. New York: Anchor Books.

———. 2001. "Apocalypse Then." Review of *Late Victorian Holocausts* by Mike Davis. *New York Times*. https://archive.nytimes.com.

Scott-Smith, Tom. 2020. *On An Empty Stomach. Two Hundred Years of Hunger Relief*. Ithaca, NY: Cornell University Press.

Sheldrake, Merlin. 2020. *Entangled Life. How Fungi Make Our Worlds, Change Our Minds & Shape Our Futures*. New York: Random House.

Steinmetz, George. 2022. "The Algerian Origins of Bourdieu's Concepts and His Rejection of Social Reproductionism." *Rassegna Italiana di Sociologia* no. 2 (April–June): 323–48.

Warde, Alan. 2016. *The Practice of Eating*. New York: Wiley.

SCOTT ALVES BARTON is a cultural anthropologist of African diaspora foodways at Notre Dame University and previously was an executive chef. Scott's research focuses on diaspora women's knowledge, intergenerational teaching/learning, cultural heritage, and political resistance in northeastern Brazil. His forthcoming manuscript, *Reckoning with Violence and Black Death*, follows *Buried in the Heart,* his exhibition on anti-Black violence, funerary foods, and ancestrality,.

AMY BENTLEY is Professor in the Department of Nutrition and Food Studies at New York University. A historian by training, her work focuses on the meanings and uses of food in the twentieth and twenty-first century United States. Publications include *Eating for Victory: Food Rationing and the Politics of Domesticity* (1998) and *Inventing Baby Food: Taste, Health, and the Industrialization of the American Diet* (2014), which was a James Beard Award finalist and an ASFS Best Book Award winner.

JENNIFER SCHIFF BERG earned her PhD in food studies at NYU. She directed the graduate food studies program since its inception in 1996 and became chair of the Department of Nutrition and Food Studies in 2023. Her research focuses on twentieth-century New York City immigration. She co-directs the NYU Urban Farm Lab.

GRACE CHOI is the founder of Larabee, an early-stage procedural knowledge company. Prior to Larabee, she taught courses in food and psychology, hosted programming for the Cooking Channel, and cooked in restaurants in New York and Italy. She resides in the Washington, DC, area with her family.

CAROLYN DIMITRI is an applied economist with a research and teaching portfolio that spans a variety of topics related to the food system, including an intensive focus on the organic food system. She is currently a member of the food studies faculty at New York University.

JONATHAN M. DEUTSCH is Professor of Culinary Arts and Science at Drexel University in Philadelphia. A certified research chef, he is director of food entrepreneurship and innovation programs, which includes the Drexel Food Lab. He earned his PhD in food studies and food Management from NYU.

JUAN C. S. HERRERA studies food consumption, food recipes, and food supply chains. He is particularly interested in understanding how these components of the food system develop over time. His methodological approach uses quantitative and qualitative methodologies such as data science, network science, econometrics, archival research, and historical methods.

ERIC HIMMELFARB is a doctoral candidate and adjunct professor in food studies at NYU. His work explores poetics as a creative and critical tool that generates movement toward, and meaning around, issues of equity and justice in the food system.

JAMES EDWARD MALIN is the engineering and science librarian for the Cooper Union for the Advancement of Science and Art and a consulting food history researcher. He is committed to serving academic communities on information literacy topics but also researches the emergence of modern food culture and its confluence with scientific understanding.

MARION NESTLE is the Paulette Goddard Professor of Nutrition, Food Studies, and Public Health at New York University, emerita, in the department she chaired from 1988 to 2003. She writes, teaches, and speaks about food politics, has written fifteen books, blogs daily (almost) at www.foodpolitics.com, and posts on X @marionnestle.

FABIO PARASECOLI is Professor of Food Studies in the Nutrition and Food Studies Department at New York University. His research explores the cultural politics of food, particularly in media, design, and heritage.

Recent books include *Food* (2019), *Global Brooklyn: Designing Food Experiences in World Cities* (2021, coedited with Mateusz Halawa), and *Gastronativism: Food, Identity, Politics* (2022).

KRISHNENDU RAY is Professor of Food Studies at NYU. He is the author of *The Migrant's Table* (2004) and *The Ethnic Restaurateur* (2016) and the coeditor of *Curried Cultures, Globalization, Food and South Asia* (2012). He is an editorial collective member of the leading food studies journal, *Gastronomica*.

STEPHANIE ROGUS is a registered dietitian and is Affiliated Faculty of Human Nutrition and Dietetic Science in the Department of Family and Consumer Sciences at New Mexico State University. She studies the economic, social, and environmental influences on food choice and impacts of food programs and policy on diet quality.

LISA SASSON is a registered dietitian and Clinical Professor at New York University's Department of Nutrition and Food Studies and Associate Dean of Global Affairs and Experiential Learning. She teaches a variety of undergraduate and graduate courses and collaborates with the NYU dental faculty to advance nutrition and oral health in the dental curriculum.

BETH C. WEITZMAN is Professor of Health and Public Policy at New York University's Steinhardt School. She has evaluated programs and policies aimed at meeting the health, social service, housing, educational, and nutritional needs of poor urban communities. Her current research focuses on calorie labels and sugar taxes.

INDEX

abductive reasoning, 147

academic disciplines, 15. *See also specific disciplines*

acarajé (black-eyed pea fritters), 56

access, 100–103; geography and, 75–76; price identifying, 62; public policy and, 71–78; racialized, 75

Accreditation Council for Education in Nutrition and Dietetics (ACEND), 104–5

Achebe, Chinua, 54

activism, 41. *See also* advocacy

additives, 100

Advanced Seminar on Food and Gender, 25

advertising. *See* marketing

advocacy, 41, 183; barriers to, 185; community and, 185; food industry opposition, 185; Nestle on, 184–86; public policy and, 33; Ray on, 186–88; standard methods for, 185; support for, 185; targets, 184–85; training, 105

aesthetics, 10. *See also* food design

affect theory, 36

Affordable Health Care Act, 79

AFHVS. *See* Agriculture, Food, and Human Values Society

agency, 183

agriculture: civic, 101; environmental impacts of, 71; greenmarkets and local, 77; history, 21; inventory-taking approach to, 45; organic, 189–91

Agriculture, Food, and Human Values Society (AFHVS), 23, 205

Albala, Ken, 126

analysis, 144

"The Anatomy of a Recipe" (Fisher), 125–26

Annales school, 6

anthropology, 6, 21, 36, 51, 152

anticolonial nationalism, 188

Appadurai, Arjun, 126

Appetite for Change (Belasco), 22–23

applied knowledge, 10, 123

applied sciences, 123

Arrighi, Giovanni, 29

ASFS. *See* Association for the Study of Food and Society

assemblage, 47

Association for the Study of Food and Society (ASFS), 22, 205

authenticity, 54–55; relativity of, 56

Avakian, Arlene Voski, 21

baby food, 24

Bachórz, Agata, 151, 192–93

banana story, 117–19

banquete sagrado da comida de santo, 52, 53, 56

Barraclough, Geoffrey, ix–x

Barthes, Roland, 29

Barton, Sylvia Pauline Alves, 50

Bates, Marcia, 174

Beasley, Myron, 60

behavioral changes: through food design, 145. *See also* diet

Belasco, Warren, 21, 22–23, 172

belonging, 95

bench science, xii–xiii

Milton Keynes UK
Ingram Content Group UK Ltd.
UKHW020304090324
439054UK00001B/28